THE PUBLIC HEALTH EFFECTS OF FOOD DESERTS

WORKSHOP SUMMARY

Paula Tarnapol Whitacre, Peggy Tsai, and Janet Mulligan, *Rapporteurs*

Food and Nutrition Board

Board on Agriculture and Natural Resources

Board on Population Health and Public Health Practice

INSTITUTE OF MEDICINE *AND*
NATIONAL RESEARCH COUNCIL
OF THE NATIONAL ACADEMIES

THE NATIONAL ACADEMIES PRESS
Washington, D.C.
www.nap.edu

THE NATIONAL ACADEMIES PRESS   500 Fifth Street, N.W.   Washington, DC 20001

NOTICE: The project that is the subject of this report was approved by the Governing Board of the National Research Council, whose members are drawn from the councils of the National Academy of Sciences, the National Academy of Engineering, and the Institute of Medicine.

This workshop was supported by Contract No. AG-3K06-C-08-0034 between the National Academy of Sciences and the U.S. Department of Agriculture. Any opinions, findings, and conclusions or recommendations in this document are those of the authors and do not necessarily reflect the views of the organizations or agencies that provided support for the project.

International Standard Book Number-13:   978-0-309-13728-7
International Standard Book Number-10:   0-309-13728-4

Additional copies of this report are available from the National Academies Press, 500 Fifth Street, N.W., Lockbox 285, Washington, DC 20055; (800) 624-6242 or (202) 334-3313 (in the Washington metropolitan area); Internet, http://www.nap.edu.

For more information about the Institute of Medicine, visit the IOM homepage at: **www.iom.edu.**

Copyright 2009 by the National Academy of Sciences. All rights reserved.

Printed in the United States of America

Cover credit: Top left: Urban corner store in Baltimore, MD, courtesy of Joel Gittelsohn. *Top right:* Fast food stock photo, with permission from iStock.com. *Bottom left:* Dollar store, courtesy of Joseph Sharkey. *Bottom right:* Enclosed urban grocery in Baltimore, MD, courtesy of Joel Gittelsohn. *Center:* Farmers market in Washington, DC, courtesy of Kamweti Mutu.

The serpent has been a symbol of long life, healing, and knowledge among almost all cultures and religions since the beginning of recorded history. The serpent adopted as a logotype by the Institute of Medicine is a relief carving from ancient Greece, now held by the Staatliche Museen in Berlin.

Suggested citation: IOM (Institute of Medicine) and National Research Council (NRC). 2009. *The public health effects of food deserts: Workshop summary*. Washington, DC: The National Academies Press.

"Knowing is not enough; we must apply.
Willing is not enough; we must do."
—Goethe

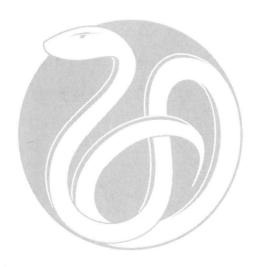

INSTITUTE OF MEDICINE
OF THE NATIONAL ACADEMIES

Advising the Nation. Improving Health.

THE NATIONAL ACADEMIES
Advisers to the Nation on Science, Engineering, and Medicine

The **National Academy of Sciences** is a private, nonprofit, self-perpetuating society of distinguished scholars engaged in scientific and engineering research, dedicated to the furtherance of science and technology and to their use for the general welfare. Upon the authority of the charter granted to it by the Congress in 1863, the Academy has a mandate that requires it to advise the federal government on scientific and technical matters. Dr. Ralph J. Cicerone is president of the National Academy of Sciences.

The **National Academy of Engineering** was established in 1964, under the charter of the National Academy of Sciences, as a parallel organization of outstanding engineers. It is autonomous in its administration and in the selection of its members, sharing with the National Academy of Sciences the responsibility for advising the federal government. The National Academy of Engineering also sponsors engineering programs aimed at meeting national needs, encourages education and research, and recognizes the superior achievements of engineers. Dr. Charles M. Vest is president of the National Academy of Engineering.

The **Institute of Medicine** was established in 1970 by the National Academy of Sciences to secure the services of eminent members of appropriate professions in the examination of policy matters pertaining to the health of the public. The Institute acts under the responsibility given to the National Academy of Sciences by its congressional charter to be an adviser to the federal government and, upon its own initiative, to identify issues of medical care, research, and education. Dr. Harvey V. Fineberg is president of the Institute of Medicine.

The **National Research Council** was organized by the National Academy of Sciences in 1916 to associate the broad community of science and technology with the Academy's purposes of furthering knowledge and advising the federal government. Functioning in accordance with general policies determined by the Academy, the Council has become the principal operating agency of both the National Academy of Sciences and the National Academy of Engineering in providing services to the government, the public, and the scientific and engineering communities. The Council is administered jointly by both Academies and the Institute of Medicine. Dr. Ralph J. Cicerone and Dr. Charles M. Vest are chair and vice chair, respectively, of the National Research Council.

www.national-academies.org

PLANNING COMMITTEE ON THE PUBLIC
HEALTH EFFECTS OF FOOD DESERTS*

BARRY M. POPKIN (*Chair*), Director, UNC Interdisciplinary Obesity Program, The Carla Smith Chamblee Distinguished Professor of Global Nutrition, School of Public Health Professor, Department of Nutrition, University of North Carolina, Chapel Hill

ANA V. DIEZ ROUX, Professor, Epidemiology Director, Center for Integrative Approaches to Health Disparities, Associate Director, Center for Social Epidemiology and Population Health, University of Michigan School of Public Health, Ann Arbor

JOEL GITTELSOHN, Associate Professor, Center for Human Nutrition, Department of International Health, Johns Hopkins University, Johns Hopkins Bloomberg School of Public Health, Baltimore, Maryland

BARBARA A. LARAIA, Assistant Professor, Division of Prevention Sciences, Department of Medicine, University of California, San Francisco

ROBIN A. McKINNON, Health Policy Specialist, Risk Factor Monitoring and Methods Branch Applied Research Program, National Cancer Institute, Rockville, Maryland

JOSEPH R. SHARKEY, Associate Professor, Social and Behavioral Health, Director, Texas Healthy Aging Research Network, Director, Program for Research in Nutrition and Health Disparities, School of Rural Public Health, Texas A&M Health Science Center, College Station, Texas

Study Staff

PEGGY TSAI, Study Director
JANET MULLIGAN, Research Associate
HEATHER BREINER, Program Associate
PAULA TARNAPOL WHITACRE, Consultant Science Writer
LINDA D. MEYERS, Food and Nutrition Board Director
ROBIN A. SCHOEN, Director, Board on Agriculture and Natural Resources

---

* Institute of Medicine and National Research Council planning committees are solely responsible for organizing the workshop, identifying topics, and choosing speakers. The responsibility for the published workshop summary rests with the workshop rapporteurs and the institution.

v

Staff

LINDA D. MEYERS, Director
GERALDINE KENNEDO, Administrative Assistant
ANTON L. BANDY, Financial Associate

Acknowledgments

This report is a product of the cooperation and contributions of the speakers and participants who attended the workshop on January 26-27, 2009. Their presentations helped to set the stage for the fruitful discussions in the sessions that followed.

This workshop summary report has been reviewed in draft form by individuals chosen for their diverse perspectives and technical expertise in accordance with procedures approved by the National Research Council's Report Review Committee. The purpose of the independent review is to provide candid and critical comments that will assist the institution in making its published report as sound as possible and to ensure that the report meets institutional standards of objectivity, evidence, and responsiveness to the study charge. The review comments and draft manuscript remain confidential to protect the integrity of the deliberative process. We wish to thank the following for their review of this report:

Alice Ammerman, Center for Health Promotion and Disease Prevention, University of North Carolina at Chapel Hill
Angela D. Liese, Center for Research in Nutrition and Health Disparities and Department of Epidemiology and Biostatistics, Arnold School of Public Health, University of South Carolina, Columbia
Diego Rose, School of Public Health & Tropical Medicine, Tulane University, New Orleans, Louisiana

Mary Story, Division of Epidemiology and Community Health,
    School of Public Health, University of Minnesota, Minneapolis
Elizabeth Tuckermanty, Cooperative State Research, Education, and
    Extension Service, United States Department of Agriculture,
    Washington, DC

Although the reviewers listed above have provided constructive comments and suggestions, they were not asked to endorse the conclusions or recommendations, nor did they see the final draft of the report before its release. The review of this report was overseen by **Dr. Eileen Kennedy,** Friedman School of Nutrition Science and Policy, Tufts University, Boston, Massachusetts. Appointed by the National Research Council and Institute of Medicine, she was responsible for making certain that an independent examination of this report was carried out in accordance with institutional procedures and that all review comments were carefully considered. Responsibility for the final content of this report rests entirely with the authors and the institutions.

Contents

Summary

The term "food desert" describes neighborhoods and communities that have limited access to affordable and nutritious foods. In the United States, those who live in urban and rural low-income neighborhoods are less likely to have access to supermarkets or grocery stores that provide healthy food choices. While many food desert studies have focused primarily on their socioeconomic determinants, less is known about their public health impacts—including the prevalence of obesity and the incidence of chronic diseases—on local populations.

As part of a year-long congressionally mandated study coordinated by the Economic Research Service (ERS) of the U.S. Department of Agriculture, the Institute of Medicine (IOM) and the National Research Council (NRC) were asked to convene a two-day workshop to understand the public health effects of food deserts. On January 26-27, 2009, workshop speakers provided presentations on how to measure and understand the extent of food deserts, their impact on individual behaviors and health outcomes in various populations, and effective ways to increase the availability of fruits and vegetables and to improve the food environment. Workshop participants also identified areas where additional research could be helpful to inform future efforts to increase the availability of affordable and nutritious foods. It was beyond the workshop's scope to examine ways to decrease access to unhealthy food options.

Although larger food stores are not the only outlets able to sell healthy food, their presence (or lack) is used as a proxy for access to healthy lower-cost food options. Using national-level data and community-level research, presenters confirmed that food deserts do exist in the United States, particularly in lower-income, inner-city and rural areas with few supermarkets and numerous smaller stores that stock very limited healthy food items such as fruits and vegetables. Mapping shows that these are also frequently areas with high rates of obesity and chronic, diet-related diseases. However, presenters emphasized that food retail is only one component of the total food environment that affects how people eat and, more fundamentally, their health. Another caveat is that the supply of healthy food will not suddenly induce people to buy and eat such food over less-healthy options, especially when relative prices of the healthier foods are high.

To better understand the public health implications of food deserts, speakers reviewed the evidence on the link between different foods and health outcomes. The research showed that the increased consumption of fruits and vegetables, whole grains, and healthy fats slows weight gain but does not reduce weight unless they are substituted for other more energy-dense foods, and it does have benefits in terms of cardiovascular disease (CVD) risk and some cancers. Consumption of sweetened beverages has doubled since 1965, and this has had a harmful effect on weight, CVD, and some cancers. Perhaps not coincidentally, the relative price of these beverages has decreased over time. The evidence linking diet to health outcomes discussed at the workshop points to the reality of the complex relationships between interventions and health outcomes, therefore there is no magic bullet for improving health and those limitations need to be kept in mind.

Research-based experiments and policy interventions to mitigate food deserts have included working with supermarket chains to determine new store sites in underserved areas, providing incentives to small-store owners to improve offerings, and encouraging the growth of farmers' markets that can improve access to fresh produce and possibly also accommodate payment with government nutrition assistance programs from the Supplemental Nutrition Assistance Program and the Special Supplemental Nutrition Program for Women, Infants, and Children.

A number of specific research needs were identified throughout the course of the workshop. These include the need for longitudinal research to track the same population over time as changes in their food environment occur, a focus on multiple outcome measures given the complexity of the food environment, and the role of price in food choice. Solving the food desert problem might not alone improve health or necessarily change what individuals eat. However, understanding where food deserts exist in the United States can provide guidance on where changes can be made to improve the availability of affordable healthy food options.

Marshaling resources to help alleviate food deserts in this context will be a step toward better health for all Americans.

This report is a summary of workshop presentations and discussions. Meeting transcripts and presentations served as the basis for the summary. The planning committee served as the organizing body for the workshop, and they identified themes for the workshop and invited speakers from the United States and the United Kingdom to address the various issues. The biographical sketches of members of the planning committee can be found in Appendix A, and the workshop agenda is found in Appendix B. Appendix C provides biographical sketches of invited speakers and moderators listed on the agenda. More than 75 stakeholders from the general public attended the workshop, and a list of those participants from the public is found in Appendix D.

The reader should be aware that the material presented here expresses the views and opinions of individuals participating in the workshop as either speakers, moderators, or audience members, and not the deliberations or conclusions of a formally constituted IOM or NRC committee. The invited speakers provided presentations based on their research or perceptions of research in the field. The purpose of the workshop was not to reach consensus on any single issue, but to gather information to inform the ERS food desert study in its report to Congress. These proceedings summarize only the statements of workshop participants and are not intended to be an exhaustive exploration of the subject matter nor a review of all empircal evidence on the topic.

1

Introduction

BACKGROUND

The term "food deserts" describes neighborhoods and communities that have limited access to affordable and nutritious foods. The term was first used in Scotland and characterized neighborhoods that can encompass many thousands of people and/or an extensive land area as defined by city blocks or square miles. In the United States, food deserts tend to be located in urban and rural low-income neighborhoods, where residents are less likely to have access to supermarkets or grocery stores that provide healthy food choices. For communities with few food retailers or supermarkets that stock little or no fresh produce, low-fat dairy, whole grains, and other healthy foods, those populations may be more likely to suffer from high rates of diabetes, cardiovascular disease, and obesity.

Research into the health implications of food deserts began in the United Kingdom in the 1990s, although economists and geographers had been studying spatial determinants of firm location, transaction costs, and differential prices of food for the poor since at least the 1960s. Sponsor representative Laurian Unnevehr, of the U.S. Department of Agriculture's Economic Research Service, pointed out in the introductory workshop session that community organizers have seen local food and food access as a powerful vehicle for social change for many decades. The study of food deserts, both here and in the United Kingdom, has since evolved to include public health researchers and practitioners, economists, planners, community activists, and others.

Researchers are looking at the effect of food deserts on health outcomes, as well as examining which interventions have the greatest potential to improve conditions.

CONGRESSIONAL MANDATE

The 2008 Farm Bill directed the U.S. Department of Agriculture (USDA) to undertake a study of food deserts in the United States to assess their incidence and prevalence, to identify characteristics and factors causing and influencing food deserts and their effect on local populations, and to provide recommendations for addressing the causes and effects. The Economic Research Service (ERS) is the lead agency on this effort and is collaborating with other agencies within USDA, such as the Food and Nutrition Service and the Cooperative State Research, Education, and Extension Service. Legislation also instructed USDA to work with other organizations, including the Institute of Medicine (IOM) and the National Research Council (NRC).

WORKSHOP ORGANIZATION

At the request of ERS, the IOM and the NRC convened a workshop to examine the public health implications of food deserts and to examine promising strategies for mitigating their impacts (see Box 1-1 for the Statement of Task). A six-person planning committee[1] was appointed by the IOM and the NRC, and biographical sketches of the planning committee are found in Appendix A. To address the Statement of Task, the planning committee developed a meeting agenda, found in Appendix B, and identified and invited experts to provide presentations at the workshop. Biographical sketches of the invited speakers and the session moderators are found in Appendix C. The workshop agenda was organized as a representative but not exhaustive overview of food deserts: It examined current research findings on the public health impacts of food deserts and explored ways to potentially mitigate those impacts.

At the January 26-27, 2009, workshop in Washington, DC, invited speakers gave presentations on how multidisciplinary approaches can be used to measure where and how food deserts occur as well as potential health impacts and strategies to ameliorate them. The invited speakers based their presentations primarily on their research or perceptions of research in the field. Speakers also addressed the common premise that increasing the availability of healthy foods will affect diet and produce health outcomes. The results of some research interventions and promis-

---

[1] The planning committee's role was limited to planning the workshop; this summary has been prepared by the workshop rapporteurs as a factual summary of what occurred.

BOX 1-1
Statement of Task

An ad hoc committee will plan and conduct a two-day workshop on the public health implications of food deserts. In this context, "food desert" is defined as a rural or urban low-income neighborhood or community with limited access to affordable and nutritious food. The workshop will include presentations and discussions that will focus on the health effects on local populations (including both adults and children) of limited access to affordable and nutritious food. Invited workshop presentations will discuss the impacts of food deserts on such outcomes as overall dietary intake (including examination of specific foods, such as fruit and vegetable consumption and intake of high-energy, low-nutrient foods); the prevalence of obesity and overweight; the existence of micronutrient deficiencies; food insecurity; and the incidence of chronic diseases associated with poor diets. In addition, presentations will cover promising strategies for mitigating the impacts of food deserts that have been suggested or implemented, or are in the planning stages. An individually authored summary of the workshop will be prepared, along with an unedited transcript of the workshop presentations.

ing policies and programs were discussed on how to alleviate problems related to the accessibility, availability, affordability, and quality of foods. More than 75 stakeholders from the general public attended the workshop, and a list of those participants is found in Appendix D.

DEFINING FOOD DESERTS

Shelly Ver Ploeg, of USDA ERS, noted that the definition of food desert contained in the Farm Bill is helpful (Box 1-2), but also raises questions. "Limited access," she said, "is not a well-defined measure: It could relate to distance, to price, and/or to time cost." "Affordable and nutritious food" is more of a continuum of foods. For example, fresh fruits and vegetables might be ideal, but frozen and canned fruits and vegetables, as well as prepared meals and food away from home, also provide nutrition and, in many situations, more practically. She also stressed that the focus of the study is on low-income *areas*, not individuals with low income who may or may not live in a food desert.

Planning committee chair Barry Popkin, of the University of North Carolina at Chapel Hill, stressed that the food people purchase in stores is but one aspect of their total food environment, a point reiterated by many presenters throughout the workshop. As noted in Figure 1-1, we eat

---

BOX 1-2
What Is a Food Desert?

In the 2008 Farm Bill, Section 7527 defines a food desert as "an area in the United States with limited access to affordable and nutritious food, particularly such an area composed of predominantly lower-income neighborhoods and communities."

In developing the framework and selected topics for this workshop, the planning committee believed it was important to specify geography and quality as factors describing a food desert and defined it more accurately as the following:

Food desert: a geographic area, particularly lower-income neighborhoods and communities, where access to affordable, quality, and nutritious foods is limited.

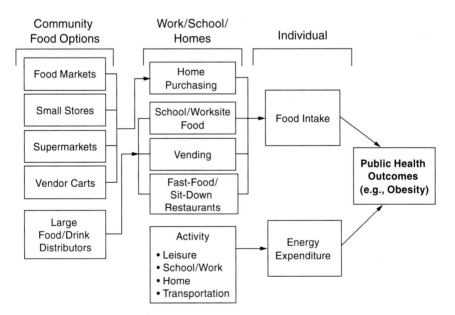

FIGURE 1-1 Causal web: role of the food environment on diet-related problems. SOURCE: B. Popkin, 2009.

in restaurants, at school, and at work. We purchase food and beverages at fast-food restaurants and from vending machines, in school cafeterias and in sit-down restaurants. Food retailers are an important piece of the puzzle, but they only contribute to one factor affecting choice in the American diet. While it was important to note the multiple aspects of the food environment to explain the how complex the issues are, Popkin reiterated that it was outside the workshop scope to address the increased access to unhealthy food options beyond the community food options setting. There is much potential for improving the situation of food deserts—providing oases of healthy food in areas without it, to extend the analogy—however, Popkin and other presenters warned against oversimplified definitions and solutions from the start of the workshop.

ORGANIZATION OF THE WORKSHOP SUMMARY

The workshop consisted of sessions discussing how food deserts can be measured (Chapter 2), the challenges and different approaches to identifying effects of the food environment on health (Chapter 3), the potential health consequences of changes in diet (Chapter 4), lessons from current intervention research to mitigate food deserts, and policy and program options that, although promising, have to date been less rigorously evaluated (Chapter 5). Many of the researchers' work cut across several themes, and the chapters are organized around presentations rather than strictly around themes. After each set of presentations within those sessions, speakers participated in moderated panel discussions with questions from the audience. In the final session of the workshop, various discussion threads mentioned by speakers and participants about additional research needed on the topic of food deserts were tied together by rapporteurs who summarized the current research gaps and future research activities necessary to fully characterize and understand the extent of food deserts and methods to address those issues (Chapter 6). This publication summarizes the presentations and discussions of the workshop.

2

Determining the Extent of Food Deserts

The food environment is a dynamic one and can change rapidly due to many factors, such as prices and preferences. To understand why food deserts are a problem and what they impact, the first session of the workshop featured presentations on the multiple dimensions used to define the food environment and the various cross-cutting ways to measure impact on both the macro and the micro levels. Lisa Powell provided a national overview and discussed price and outlet availability as aspects of access to healthy food. Mari Gallagher focused on the urban environments in Chicago and Detroit, while Joseph Sharkey pointed out the changing food retail environment in rural Brazos Valley, Texas. Lastly, Ephraim Leibtag discussed the dynamics of the food shopping environment and how it affects access to affordable and healthy foods.

NATIONAL OVERVIEW OF FOOD DESERTS BY DEMOGRAPHICS AND SOCIOECONOMIC STATUS

Lisa M. Powell, of the University of Illinois at Chicago, presented national data categorized by U.S. zip codes to provide a bird's eye view of areas that do not have access to a supermarket or a grocery store. In doing so, she acknowledged that there is a trade-off between using data available on a national level versus the greater detail available from onsite data collection across smaller geographic areas.

Access to healthy foods means that the food is available and affordable. Powell defined availability as the number of food-related outlets within a measured geographic area assessed on a per capita and/or a per land area basis, with healthy foods associated with grocery store and supermarket availability and less-healthy foods associated with convenience store and fast-food restaurant availability. Availability gets at the time costs associated with food shopping (e.g., a convenience store that is a five-minute walk away versus a supermarket that is a half-hour bus ride away), whereas affordability is the monetary cost or purchase price of various items. Based on their available price data, the affordability of healthy foods is represented by the prices of fruits and vegetables and of less-healthy foods by the prices of fast food and soft drinks. Taken together, Powell mentioned that availability and affordability determine the total cost of food, or its accessibility.

To provide an overview of accessibility, Powell and her team use data from the American Chamber of Commerce Researchers Association (ACCRA) for food prices and from Dun and Bradstreet (D&B) for outlet density. Drawing on D&B data, supermarkets and grocery stores are distinguished from convenience stores by the assumption that access to a convenience store alone does not provide access to quality food. Supermarkets are substantially larger food stores than grocery stores and are more likely to have onsite food preparation such as a butcher, a baker, and a deli. Chain stores are studied because they often benefit from economies of scale in terms of purchasing power, distribution, and other factors that contribute to lower prices. A validation study is under way to ensure that the outlet data available from D&B and infoUSA, another proprietary business database, do not contain biases across neighborhoods of different socioeconomic status and racial or ethnic characteristics.

Availability

Using D&B data, 29 percent of zip codes nationwide do not have a grocery store or supermarket, and 74 percent do not have a chain supermarket. Powell stressed that using zip codes alone is misleading, given that some zip codes contain no or very few people, and therefore she narrowed in on more densely populated urban areas. Of these urban areas, 7 percent have no grocery store or supermarket and 53 percent do not have a chain supermarket.

When her team looked at food availability by linking D&B data in 28,050 zip codes with U.S. Census data on race, ethnicity, income, population, and degree of urbanization for the year 2000 (Powell et al., 2007), based on multivariate models, quite significant differences emerged:

- African-American populations had half as much access to chain supermarkets as Caucasians, controlling for other factors;

- Hispanic populations had one-third the access to chain supermarkets as non-Hispanics, controlling for other factors;
- Lower-income neighborhoods overall had less access to chain stores than middle- and upper-income neighborhoods; and
- Independent, non-chain stores were more prevalent in predominantly African-American and Hispanic communities than in predominantly Caucasian communities.

As observed throughout the workshop, longitudinal data on various aspects of research on food deserts are scarce. However, Powell has done some national-level comparisons of changes in food availability in 1997 versus 2008. Looking at predominantly African-American (defined as 70 percent and higher), predominantly Caucasian (70 percent and higher), and mixed neighborhoods, the predominantly African-American neighborhoods had the smallest increase in overall availability and the largest decrease in number of grocery stores since 1997. When looked at by income, lower-income neighborhoods had the smallest growth in overall access to food stores and the largest decrease in number of grocery stores (Figure 2-1).

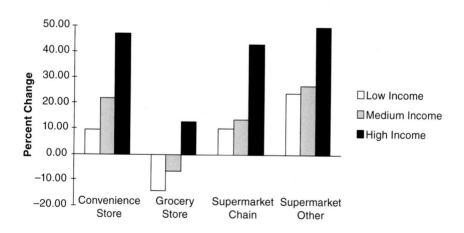

FIGURE 2-1 Change in food store availability by income, 1997-2008.
SOURCE: Lisa M. Powell, ImpacTeen Project, University of Illinois at Chicago.
Data drawn from Dun & Bradstreet, 1997 and 2008.

Affordability

Real (inflation-adjusted) prices for fruits and vegetables, dairy, and meat were generally flat from 1990 through 2007, based on ACCRA data. Yet, over the same period, real prices for soft drinks and fast foods—as noted earlier, the proxies for less-healthy foods—declined significantly (soft drinks by one-third, fast food by 12 percent), making them seem increasingly less expensive relative to healthier alternatives. Powell noted that people operate in terms of relative prices, so it has become relatively cheaper over time to purchase energy-dense foods such as fast food items like burgers and fries.

Powell and Bao (in press) recently linked price and outlet density data with longitudinal data from 1998 through 2002 on the children of mothers from the 1979 National Longitudinal Survey of Youth. They found that food pricing is likely to have modest but measurable effects on weight outcomes of children ages 6 to 17 and that greater access to supermarkets, when defined on a per land area basis, is associated with a reduction in weight. Price elasticities were stronger for children in families of lower socioeconomic status: for example, among children in the bottom quintile of the income distribution, a 10 percent reduction in the prices of fruits and vegetables was associated with a 1.4 percent reduction in body mass index and a 10 percent increase in fast food prices was associated with a 2.6 percent reduction. This evidence, she concluded, suggests a multi-pronged approach of changing relative prices by both subsidizing fruits and vegetables and taxing fast food to improve weight outcomes among children and adolescents.

MEASURING FOOD DESERTS: FOCUSING ON URBAN AREAS

Mari Gallagher, of Mari Gallagher Research & Consulting Group, helped create the nonprofit National Center for Public Research. Through that group, she and others focus their research efforts on food deserts, and she presented findings from work in Chicago and Detroit. Gallagher pointed out that there are untrue stereotypes about food deserts—that food deserts only affect inner-city, African-American, or poor people—and these false notions may discourage investment by retailers.

Gallagher differentiated between two different types of food venues: mainstream and fringe. Mainstream food venues are grocery stores or supermarkets, both small and large, where healthy foods can be purchased. On the other hand, Gallagher mentioned that fringe food venues—including fast-food restaurants, gas stations, and convenience and liquor stores—do not have healthy food options available on a regular basis. A community will usually have both types of food venues. The key, however, is a term Gallagher calls *food balance*, so that consumers can easily choose between a mainstream or a fringe food store. A food balance score is a ratio of the distance to the closest grocer versus distance to the closest fringe food establishment. When fringe food venues are handy but mainstream stores are not, a community is out of balance.

Food Balance Effect

Gallagher and her associates derive a food balance score for a neighborhood, then pair a food balance score with health-outcome data. To determine food balance, they conduct block-level analyses to find the location of the closest grocer and fast-food (since modified to fringe food) establishment, which they then pair with tract-level data on diet-related deaths. A food balance score reflects the fact that there is no perfect distance to a grocery store, given the different characteristics of different markets such as transportation options and geography. Rather, a food balance score gets around these characteristics to provide a relative measurement.

Using these methods in Chicago, three key food deserts became evident, comprising about 500,000 people and the city's highest concentration of single mothers and children. These areas were the most "out of balance," using the definition above, with fringe food far closer than mainstream venues, especially for majority African-American areas (see Figure 2-2).

Residents of food deserts face nutritional challenges evident in diet-related community health outcomes. Gallagher stated that her unpublished research shows communities with out-of-balance food environments having statistically significant higher rates of residents' dying prematurely from diabetes, when income, education, and race are controlled for. Gallagher found that African-American communities are most likely to experience the greatest total years of life lost from diabetes as a result. Furthermore, through an analysis of body mass index (BMI) based on drivers' license data in Chicago, the areas with the highest BMI are roughly the same areas indicated as food deserts. Gallagher's unpublished regression analysis shows that opening in a grocery store has a better impact on reducing obesity than closing a fast-food restaurant.

In Detroit, the team studied 50,000 blocks and found that very few had mainstream grocery stores. They more likely had various types of convenience or fringe stores, particularly liquor or party stores that sell a few food items along with cigarettes, alcohol, and soft drinks. In some cases, some of the fringe outlets were classified as grocery stores in USDA data, which the team recoded after visiting the establishments. After this recoding of 1,300 retailers that accept USDA Food Stamps in the Detroit neighborhoods studied, 92 percent were fringe retailers, including liquor

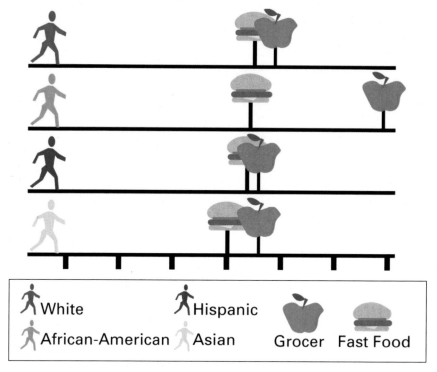

FIGURE 2-2 Relative distance to grocers and fast food in Chicago.
SOURCE: M. Gallagher, 2009.

stores, party stores, gas stations, and buy-and-fry shops, and only 8 percent, or fewer than 100, were grocery stores of any size.

The Role of Convenience

Gallagher asserted that people generally buy food at the places closest to them, even if the stores do not have the foods they may prefer or need. Thus, concentrating on the price, quality, and range of healthy food choices in existing locations is important. In her opinion, a store that "crosses" from a mainstream to a fringe store, or vice versa, has a big impact on a community, since nearby shoppers may rely on it for their primary food source. Similarly, the addition or removal of a new store is significant, especially a mainstream grocery store. For example, after the Chicago study was completed, a Food 4 Less opened in the community of Englewood, one of the food deserts identified. Returning to the block-by-block analysis, the addition of the new store improved the food balance effect for more than 40,000 people, including almost 14,000 children.

Gallagher said her data raised interest among Chicago officials and supermarket executives. The data showed where in the city the impact of a new store would be greatest and, thus, helped the city prioritize six sites for grocer recruitment and incentives. The grocery representatives she has spoken with were intrigued by the possibilities of locating in underserved areas. However, they were also worried about the spotlight on food deserts because they were concerned about being swayed by political concerns for the poor. Data on food deserts could ease some of those concerns and be helpful for decision making and useful in developing policy to alleviate food access disparities.

MEASURING FOOD DESERTS: FOCUSING ON RURAL AREAS

Joseph R. Sharkey, of Texas A&M University, suggested that while each rural area is different, a study of food access in the six rural counties of Texas's Brazos Valley can be helpful to understand food deserts in rural America. The sparser population and lack of public transportation mean that low income and lack of a vehicle—or in the case of some seniors, the inability to drive their vehicles—complicate access to a store with healthy foods.

Rural Shopping Options

Borrowing from healthcare access literature (Khan and Bhardwaj, 1994; Guagliardo, 2004), Sharkey said potential consumers make decisions about where and what food to buy based on many factors. He introduced a conceptual model of food access that considers the food environment (including stores' location, price, quality, and availability) combined with consumer variables (including their own food preferences, income, transportation options, and other factors) that together determine the barriers or facilitators to healthful eating. In many rural areas, including the six Texas counties, the food environment is rapidly changing. In addition to more traditional supermarkets and grocery stores, supercenters (such as Super Wal-Mart and Super Kmart) are expanding into rural areas. These supercenters are very large stores that engage in retailing a general line of groceries in combination with general lines of merchandise. Convenience stores, or food marts, are including more food items in their product selection. Nontraditional food stores, such as mass merchandisers (including Wal-Mart, Target, and Kmart), dollar stores, and chain pharmacies are entering the food business. In Brazos Valley and other rural counties, these places are often in central locations, such as along a highway, to reach the maximum number of shoppers.

The counties studied by Sharkey and his team span 4,500 square miles and 101 census block groups. There are five small urban clusters and no public transportation. To observe the location of food stores and the availability of fresh or processed fruits and vegetables, they drove all the major roads and conducted in-store surveys of food items available in all traditional, convenience, and nontraditional food stores. Residents' mean distance to a supermarket is 9.9 miles, with grocery, convenience, and nontraditional stores somewhat closer. Most neighborhoods do not have any type of food store within a mile, but for those that do, the store is most likely a convenience store.

Rural Access to Fruits and Vegetables: Fresh and Processed

Different types of stores offer a range of fresh and processed (canned or frozen) fruits and vegetables. Supermarkets, supercenters, and grocery stores offer fresh produce, while convenience and nontraditional food stores, with few exceptions, offer only canned fruits and vegetables. To access fresh fruits and vegetables, about one-third of the population must travel 10 miles or more, although that percentage is halved if processed food is included (see Figures 2-3 and 2-4).

The residents who live in urban clusters—about 25 percent of the total population in five clusters of between 3,500 and 11,950 people—are among the most socioeconomically deprived households in the Brazos Valley. Even in these five towns, there is limited access by walking and there is no public transportation. Thus, these residents have difficulty accessing healthy food.

Sharkey summed up what his research in the Brazos Valley shows about food deserts in rural areas: Access is particularly problematic for rural residents without vehicles or sufficient financial resources. Most rural neighborhoods are not near supermarkets or even smaller stores that stock fruits and vegetables. As elsewhere, store formats are changing, with superstores, convenience stores, dollar stores, and even pharmacies getting into the food business. The older population, with more limited mobility, is increasing. Sharkey said that these factors from his model of food access suggest focusing efforts on stores that people currently use, the frequency with which they shop, and the types of products they purchase.

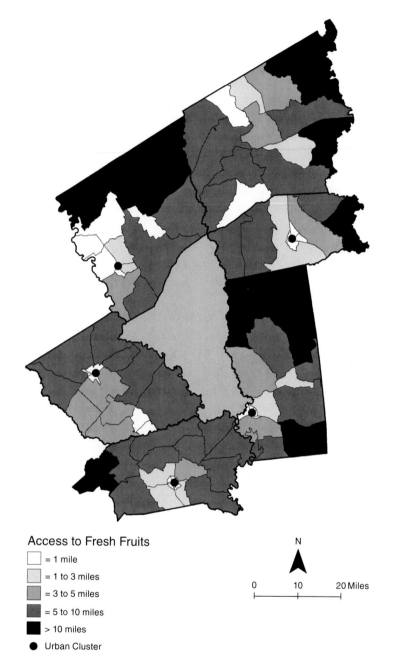

FIGURE 2-3 Access to fresh fruits by distance to nearest vendor.
SOURCE: Sharkey, 2009.

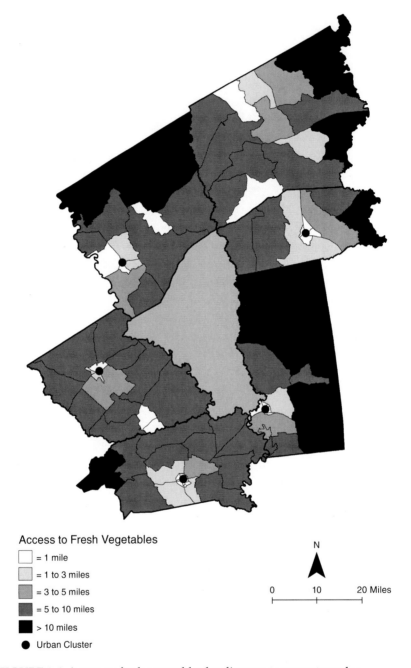

FIGURE 2-4 Access to fresh vegetables by distance to nearest vendor.
SOURCE: Sharkey, 2009.

DYNAMICS OF THE FOOD SHOPPING ENVIRONMENT

To provide a national perspective, Ephraim Leibtag, of the U.S. Department of Agriculture's Economic Research Service, summarized government and proprietary data to discuss current trends in the retail food environment. The government data include producer and consumer price information from the Bureau of Labor Statistics and geocoding of store locations from the Census of Retail Trade. Consumer-based data include the Consumer Expenditure Survey, American Time Use Survey, and National Health and Nutrition Examination Survey. Nielsen's Scan-track and Information Resources, Inc.'s Infoscan databases track store sales for major grocery store chains, while consumer shopping and eating information can be analyzed using the NPD Group's National Eating Trends and Consumer Reports on Eating Share Trends data along with Nielsen's Homescan data. Neighborhood and local economies were not discussed in this presentation on the national overview.

Price Stability and Volatility

After a relatively stable period of 20 years, when prices were flat or even falling in real terms, commodity prices spiked in 2008, with most basic food crops and energy costs at record highs. However, with the recession, prices fell in late 2008-early 2009. One legacy of price stability was the advantage of mass production, in which suppliers centralized operations to set up large distribution chains.

Three of the main factors that determine retail food prices are the costs of goods sold and operating costs, the dynamics of competition in the market, and consumer demand. Almost 40 percent of every dollar that a consumer spends on food goes for labor, with less than 20 percent going to the agricultural sector and the rest for expenses that range from advertising to rent to energy (see Figure 2-5).

Until the late 1980s, the Consumer Price Index for food and the Producer Price Index for finished consumer foods tracked closely, and traditional food retailers were by far the dominant players in the marketplace. Comparing these indices in the past two decades explains why the retail environment has become more crowded. As the indices diverged, with consumer prices rising faster than producer prices, new types of retailers saw a business opportunity—and joined traditional grocery stores and supermarkets in selling food to consumers.

The Rise of Nontraditional Retailers

As recently as 1998, grocery stores and supermarkets accounted for 80 percent of the consumer food dollar. Nontraditional stores now get 40

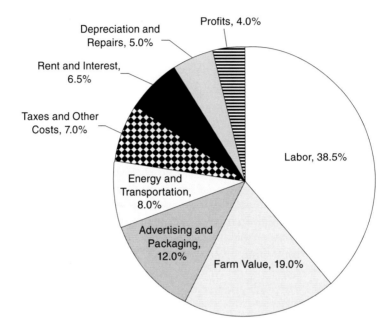

FIGURE 2-5 Breakdown of a consumer dollar spent on food.
SOURCE: Leibtag, 2009.

percent of Americans' food dollars, and the percentage has been increasing. For example, in 2003, about 1,000 Wal-Mart Supercenters operated around the country; by 2008, that number had more than doubled to 2,400. Traditional stores are squeezed in the middle and are trying to determine their niche. Wal-Mart and warehouse stores offer lower prices and large quantities. Dollar and other discount stores offer a more limited item assortment, have lower expenses than some supermarkets, and oftentimes focus on selling to low-income households. Meanwhile, gourmet and organic stores target more upscale consumers.

The traditional retailers must figure out their niche and determine optimum size in terms of scale and efficiency. As Leibtag observed, a "plain old grocery store does not really cut it anymore." Retailers are looking to distinguish themselves in terms of price, special items such as organic produce or fresh meats, or other characteristics. Some are building smaller stores that are more amenable to urban locations.

Overall consumer food prices rose 5.5 percent in 2008, which was the largest increase since 1990. Although prices have declined from their record highs, the situation remains uncertain, increasing the difficulty of making predictions about the retailing environment. Yet it seems evident that the more competitive diversity of stores selling food and the wider range of consumer food options are not going to change any time soon.

DISCUSSION: MEASURING FOOD DESERTS

Heidi Blanck, of the Centers for Disease Control and Prevention, moderated the discussion period after the speakers' presentations. The questions were submitted by workshop participants invited from the general public. Many questions centered on data collection and the most effective ways to interpret and use the available data.

Prices and Child BMI

Several questions centered on the effects of fruit and vegetable prices on children's weight. Powell explained how her research linked price and outlet density data by geocodes with individual-level data to examine relationships between these economic contextual factors and food consumption behavior and weight outcomes. Higher prices for fruits and vegetables are expected to decrease consumption of these foods and increase weight. She cautioned against assuming that the presence of a supermarket that sells healthier food will always lead to better diets, especially without taking account of prices. Whereas cross-sectional models rely on comparisons across different people, a longitudinal framework examines the same individuals over time, which helps to disentangle causal relationships.

Sharkey noted that the variety of items stocked in stores poses a challenge to research into the effect of price on consumption. Meaningful comparisons are difficult when stores carry different items, although agricultural economists at his institution are attempting to devise common measures. He also suggested that the access point for food shopping, in many cases, is not where people live, but where they work or engage in other daily activities.

Gallagher shared findings from two focus groups of participants who live far from mainstream grocers, with one group slightly better off economically. She said both groups were distance-sensitive, but much more price-sensitive. They desired different fruits and vegetables, but, she said, "they were pretty much price shopping all the time."

Role of Qualitative Research

Most panelists agreed that more qualitative research is needed, in which people living in food deserts describe their access and how it might impact their food choices. For example, Gallagher said even the

---

BOX 2-1
Listening and Learning

In addition to understanding how socioeconomic and demographic determinants impact food deserts, it is important that qualitative research also consider other contextual factors that influence people and their food choices. For example, a low-income mother was concerned about her teenage son's unscheduled time after school and contracted with him to come home after school to care for a younger sibling. He agreed if his friends could also come over. His mother soon found that an unexpected consequence was that she had to provide snacks to a group of hungry teenage boys. The economic imperative favored providing them with energy-dense snacks. In this case, a mother with limited resources needed to address child-care needs while balancing the household food budget. The bottom line is that it is imperative to link quantitative data with the context of people's lives because socioeconomic factors are interconnected with other variables that may be overlooked.

---

quickly organized focus groups mentioned above highlighted that the respondents would not welcome a grocery delivery service, because of bad experiences with spoiled or rotten food purchased from local stores, whereas an outsider might have considered such a service a viable option. Powell said her team used focus groups to conduct qualitative research with adolescents in terms of when and what they ate during the day. Sharkey incorporates quantitative and qualitative methods, such as observing participants within their own homes. It is imperative, he said, especially when policy decisions are in the mix, to link quantitative data with an understanding of the context in which people live (Box 2-1).

Agglomeration of Stores

A topic touched on in this panel, and returned to throughout the workshop, is what Gallagher termed the agglomeration of stores: "Grocers do not go where grocers do not go already," with the converse being true as well. One concern often expressed is that a supercenter will drive out other stores. In contrast, Gallagher's research in urban areas has shown that businesses thrive when they are located near each other, and in fact, other retailers do well in locations near supercenters. The highest level of retail helps shape the environment of the commercial district, which is why a proliferation of fringe stores will discourage a more mainstream store from entering a market.

Consumer Shopping Patterns

A member of the audience noted that the presence of a supermarket provides access to healthier options, but it also increases access to lower-cost, energy-dense or "junk" foods. Gallagher said the Food 4 Less that opened in Chicago has found it difficult to sell some healthier foods, such as low-fat versus whole milk. Powell reminded the group that the mere presence of a store may not change consumption patterns and related weight outcomes if unhealthy energy-dense foods are substantially cheaper than healthy less-energy-dense foods. Observing what is inside customers' shopping carts confirms that they often buy less-healthy foods, both because of price and because they have tastes that have developed for many years. Supply and demand must match up: the food must be on the shelf, but people have to buy it. Blanck added that product placement within stores can also help influence decisions.

In reply to a question about whether different racial or ethnic sub-groups have different kinds of stores they prefer, Leibtag said the work he has seen on this topic does not show a large difference—people usually shop close to where they live—although there are differences in shopping behavior by demographic group. Unless a tax or subsidy were extreme, he does not think it would alter food choice by much, because of taste preferences. Gallagher suggested there might be an opportunity to tighten the rules of inclusion for Supplemental Nutrition Assistance Program (SNAP; formerly known as the federal Food Stamp Program) retailers so that participating outlets will have to offer healthier foods. However, she warned about some pushback, as residents expressed concern that fringe food retailers would shut down or stop accepting SNAP vouchers if rules were too stringent.

Using Data in Policy Making

Gallagher mentioned that many organizations around the country, such as the Chicago Food Policy Advisory Council, have done excellent work providing data for policy formation. Regular tracking helps direct limited resources. As she noted, "We need to keep the data honest, keep it live, and make sure that we are looking at the full picture of what is going on and not just certain neighborhoods." In terms of presenting data, maps have been most useful in informing policy makers and the public about the scope of the situation.

Population and Economic Changes

Referring to Powell's presentation about store growth over the last decade, a participant asked whether population decline in low-income or underserved neighborhoods might be the reason behind the less vigorous growth of stores. Powell had used 2000 census data and will update the information when new census figures are available. However, she said she did not think this was a significant factor except perhaps for cases on the margin.

As the recession deepens, local employment will be affected and customers may purchase more energy-dense, relatively cheaper foods. Some stores, including food outlets, will go out of business or curtail services. In that regard, said Gallagher, two food stores in close proximity to each other can keep the market competitive and this would benefit consumers. In contrast, a store without competition, faced with dwindling profit margins, may not maintain cleanliness and service, thus exacerbating its problems.

3

Studying Food Deserts Through Different Lenses

The food environment is complex, as are people's decisions about where to live and shop, and what to buy and eat. As discussed in Chapter 2, the availability of healthy foods affects food choice, but supply alone does not guarantee that healthier foods will be purchased, especially by price-conscious shoppers. Presenters in the next session looked at food deserts with some complementary methodological approaches—epidemiology, geography, and economics and urban planning—and discussed what they can and cannot tell us about the link between food access and health.

EPIDEMIOLOGICAL APPROACH

As researchers investigate ways to improve people's health, they have turned to the local food environment. Ana Diez Roux, of the University of Michigan, described aspects of the food environment as "features of the local physical environment that facilitate the consumption of certain types of foods and detract from the consumption of others." She suggested several health-related reasons for this approach:

- Focusing exclusively on individuals, without taking account of their surrounding environment, has led to disappointing results;
- Neighborhoods serve as the context for physical and social exposures that may be related to health;
- Neighborhoods may have causal effects and/or constraints on prevention efforts; and

- Neighborhood differences, including race, ethnicity, and socioeconomic factors, may contribute to health inequalities and have public health and policy relevance.

Space as a Health Determinant

Space—as defined by place, neighborhood, or environment—is a key dimension across which health is patterned. For example, there is a five-fold difference in diabetes prevalence rates across New York City neighborhoods, according to calculations by the New York City Department of Health & Mental Hygiene, the U.S. Centers for Disease Control and Prevention, and the World Health Organization. These differences could occur because residents are segregated by factors that research has shown are health-related (such as income, race, or ethnic group), but the features of the places themselves may contribute to the problem. However, Diez Roux emphasized that environmental constraints and reinforcements, such as local food availability and affordability, are just some of many factors that affect health.

As discussed by the previous panel, researchers have used many different databases and instruments to understand local food environments. Two important points emerged: (1) the local food environment is patterned by areas of socioeconomic, race, and ethnic composition; and (2) features of the local food environment have been cross-sectionally associated with the diet of residents and with related health outcomes. In an ancillary study of the Multiethnic Study of Atherosclerosis (MESA), in which Diez Roux was the principal investigator, supermarkets were less common in low-income areas, and liquor stores and small grocery stores were more common (Moore and Diez Roux, 2006). The smaller stores did not stock many healthy foods. Moreover, even supermarket offerings can vary by location. A comparison of two supermarkets—one in predominantly African-American Baltimore City and one in predominantly Caucasian Baltimore County—showed that the inner-city store offered far fewer healthy options (see Table 3-1).

A Gap: Longitudinal Studies and Better Understanding of Causality

How do these differences in food availability relate to health outcomes? Studies show that respondents living in neighborhoods with the lowest availability of healthy food, as indicated by surveys of residents or lower density of supermarkets, were 32 to 55 percent less likely to have a good-quality diet than those with greater availability (Moore et al., 2008). In addition, measures of the availability of healthy food in stores are also related to the diet of residents (Franco et al., 2009). Diez Roux stressed that

TABLE 3-1 Healthy Food Availability Index, Comparing Two Supermarkets

Location:	Baltimore City		Baltimore County	
Racial composition:	97% African American		93% Caucasian	
Median household income:	$20,833		$57,391	
Foods	Availability	Points	Availability	Points
Skim milk	Yes	2	Yes	3
Fruits	17	2	59	4
Vegetables	38	3	74	4
Lean meat	No	2	Yes	3
Frozen foods	No	0	Yes	3
Low-sodium foods	No	0	Yes	2
100% whole wheat bread	Yes	2	Yes	4
Low-sugar cereals	Yes	2	Yes	2
Modified NEMS-S (0-27)		18		25

NOTE: NEMS-S = Nutrition Environment Measures Survey in stores.
SOURCE: Franco et al., 2008.

research has focused mostly on cross-sectional data, comparing different people living in different neighborhoods. A great need is longitudinal evidence relating changes in healthy food availability to changes in diet over time.

A few longitudinal studies have taken place, even though causality is not yet clear. For example, using MESA data, people who live in neighborhoods with higher healthy food availability scores had a 45 percent reduced incidence of diabetes over a five-year period (Auchincloss et al., unpublished). Another study (Sturm and Datar, 2005, 2008) confirmed that higher prices of fruits and vegetables were linked to greater increases in children's weight over time. In the Moving to Opportunity study of families who had moved from poor to non-poor neighborhoods (Kling et al., 2007), BMI was significantly reduced, although the reasons for this are not understood. Also, as discussed further in this chapter and in Chapter 5, "natural experiments" occurred in Glasgow and Leeds in the United Kingdom, where supermarkets opened in public housing areas and the areas could be studied before and after.

Challenges to understanding the causal links remain, including determining which aspects of the local food environment (e.g., availability, price, convenience) are most relevant to health, how to measure and what to use as a proxy, the scale at which changes to the local food environment are most effective, and reasonable time lags and critical periods in which to expect any effects to occur. In addition, dynamic processes are involved because just as healthy food availability may impact dietary patterns, the diets of residents may impact the kinds of foods that are available. The complex and dynamic nature of these processes means that multiple kinds of evidence will be needed to identify the best strategies for intervention, said Diez Roux. These might include improved observational studies and qualitative research, evaluation of natural experiments, and dynamic simulation approaches. Ultimately, it may be necessary to act based on the best available evidence and then rigorously evaluate the impact of these actions so that they can be improved or modified.

Diez Roux concluded by stressing why it is worth focusing on locations. Place-based and individual inequalities are mutually reinforcing, and neighborhood differences that result from specific polices are amenable to intervention. Ultimately, the goal is not just to understand causation, but to facilitate change for health and non-health benefits. The new paradigm is an interdisciplinary one and integrates transportation, urban planning, food access, and community development policies as part of dealing with people's health.

GEOSPATIAL APPROACH

Steven Cummins, of Queen Mary, University of London, brought a geographic perspective to the food desert discussion, given that space, place, and distance are features that may affect the food environment and thus become determinants of diet and health. Research into food access began in the 1960s, stemming from concern about social disparities in access to basic services, rather than from the perspective of health. In the 1990s, he said, residents in a deprived urban housing scheme in west Scotland coined the term "food desert" to describe the lack of access to a healthy, reasonably priced food supply. During this period, food stores were leaving urban centers for outlying areas, resulting in fewer, larger stores concentrated in edge-of-town sites (see Figure 3-1). A recent systematic review of 48 studies from 1966 through 2007 (Beaulac et al., in press) shows equivocal findings about the existence of food deserts in many European countries—but clear evidence of disparities in food access in the United States by income and race.

Natural Experiments

The underlying conceptual model behind why food deserts affect health is that of "deprivation amplification": Residents of low-income neighborhoods are exposed to poor-quality local food environments that amplify their individual risk factors for poor health (Macintyre, 2007). Exposure to these environments may contribute to the development of

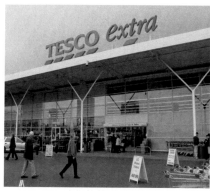
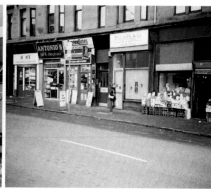

FIGURE 3-1 Comparison of two urban food environments: Springburn and Shettleston, Glasgow, 1 mile apart.
SOURCE: S. Cummins, 2009.

socioeconomic and spatial inequalities in diet-related diseases, such as obesity, diabetes, and heart disease.

The opening of two large supermarkets in Glasgow and Leeds, both in deprived areas in the United Kingdom, provided the opportunity to study the effect of increasing access to food retail opportunities as a solution (the Leeds study was discussed by Neil Wrigley during the second day of the workshop and is summarized in Chapter 5). In Glasgow, a large Tesco supermarket was opened in an area of multiple deprivation with high concentrations of public housing and very few food options.

Cummins reported that the Glasgow Superstore Study (Cummins et al., 2005) did not show that the new store resulted in positive impacts on healthy food consumption. Although disappointed with the findings of a study that had obvious intuitive policy appeal, he has since sought to understand why these negative results occurred. Follow-up qualitative work revealed community behaviors that had not been revealed through surveys. For example, some residents purposefully chose not to shop at the new store out of concern that they would be tempted to spend too much. Additionally, what constitutes "local" was clearly different for different people, whose spatial behaviors are affected by their daily routines. For instance, some people had always preferred to shop in other neighborhoods, perhaps where they had grown up, previously lived, or worked, and thus continued to do so.

Understanding what drives spatial behavior is of paramount importance in strengthening causal inference. Instead of just focusing on the supply side, Cummins stated that researchers need also to focus on demand and the geographic choices that people make that shape their health behaviors. Learning what does not work also provides valuable lessons.

Systems approaches may further understanding of food deserts and public health. The spatial patterning of health as an outcome could be conceived as an emergent property of a complex system incorporating both demand- and supply-side behaviors. Individuals affect and are affected by the environment around them in a complex dynamic system. Spatial microsimulation tools can help model and predict the effect of system change, rather than just describing it, if they are based on a solid theoretical framework. For example, Cummins has been involved in developing a spatial microsimulation model to predict the spatial patterning of diabetes changes due to age in Leeds. The next step is to try to predict what would happen to future diabetes prevalence if plausible, policy-relevant, contextual factors were modified.

Better theories are required to inform better empirical research to elucidate causal processes and predict the public health effects of food deserts. Multiple approaches and methods, including better-quality basic theory and data, qualitative methods, natural experiments, and simulations, can help triangulate the evidence base and provide a fuller picture. Better understanding of spatial behaviors harnessed to advanced spatial methods will allow the development of possible levers for environmental interventions.

ECONOMIC APPROACH

One critique of cross-sectional studies linking food access to health outcomes is that those studies do not account for access as a factor; residents choose where they live and are not randomly assigned to neighborhoods. Yan Song, of the University of North Carolina at Chapel Hill, presented perspectives from economics and urban planning as a third way to look at the food environment. Urban economics looks at issues of selectivity in how residents choose where to live, and could help explain links of food access to consumption and health outcomes. Urban planning has established principles about the mix between retail and commercial space, which can include the food environment. Song focused on how retail food outlets affect choices of where residents locate.

Since the 1960s, economists have used hedonic price models and discrete choice models to explain residential location choice, focusing on characteristics related to housing and the surrounding community. Little research has been done on how food access may enter into people's choices, although new urbanism or smart growth, in which a mixture of land uses are located in the same neighborhood within walking distance, would include food outlets.

Hedonic Price Model

A hedonic model examines the individual value-added factors in the total price of an item, such as the convenience of a residence to stores or work locations. This approach enables a researcher to identify the marginal price of any given feature, potentially including the location or size of food establishments. Research into how people value mixed-use development shows a positive price premium for having a neighborhood café and a walkable network of stores: about $6,500 in one study in Portland, Oregon (Song and Knapp, 2003, 2004; Song and Sohn, 2007). A negative premium was attached to commercial uses not in scale with the rest of the neighborhood, including big box stores.

Discrete Choice Model

In the discrete choice model, people are presumed to make a choice from a fixed set of alternatives. They decide where to live based on their own household's characteristics and the characteristics of potential dwellings. Is the food environment one of these characteristics? At this point, Song is not aware of any published studies on food environment as a factor in residential choice.

Urban Planning and Food Environments

Song explained that planners distinguish between basic, revenue-generating land use and nonbasic, service-related land use. The current curriculum at urban planning schools favors planning small-scale food stores in mixed-use development for easy access by local households. Economies of scale, consumer preferences, and existing zoning ordinances, however, can make this goal unrealistic.

In summary, the research on food environment and residential selection activity shows evidence of a price premium associated with healthy neighborhood stores, but these premiums have been observed only in high-income neighborhoods. No study has explicitly looked at how food retailers affect residential location choice. More refined surveys and more data, including natural experiments, may provide some answers.

DISCUSSION: DIFFERENT APPROACHES

Jill Reedy, of the National Cancer Institute at the National Institutes of Health, moderated the discussion that followed this panel. Many of the questions and comments related to the complexity of causes, making it difficult to separate the impact of the food environment from other variables.

Food Access from the Workplace

The research on food deserts looks at access from where people live versus where they work. One workshop participant said opposition by institutional review boards makes it difficult to collect data from workplaces. In any event, Diez Roux cautioned against extrapolating too much from a current situation: people might buy food closer to work, for example, because there is no alternative closer to home. Some groups are combining data on a variety of aspects of the built environment, including food venues and their relationship to transportation routes, to see how they connect.

Supermarkets as One Proxy

Song was asked about the emphasis on large supermarkets from a planning perspective, given the emphasis on keeping buildings at a similar scale. She observed that spatial planning may not take household characteristics sufficiently into account. Cummins said that what planners want and what a local population wants might diverge. Often a successful local retail economy has a mix of different-sized stores. Diez Roux stressed the issue is access to healthy foods, not necessarily access to a supermarket. Environments have many features that interrelate, which implies thinking through the positive and adverse effects of a particular intervention.

Role of Simulations

Simulations are valuable, said Diez Roux, because they require thinking through processes to create a valid model and may point out knowledge gaps that may have been overlooked by other research methods. Cummins noted that simulations can utilize existing observational data in a better way, perhaps linking together unconnected data sets. Song noted that in urban planning, simulations are used to build scenarios to observe the effect, holding everything else constant, of a specific policy intervention.

Mixed Land Use

Whether mixed land use promotes positive health effects is, according to Song, a debatable topic. It seems to depend on what the mixed uses actually entail. If they are appropriate and decrease automobile use, that would be healthy. Diez Roux said the literature is difficult to summarize because the measures have been so different. Proximity of destinations promotes walking, but the long-term health impacts are less known.

Realistic Expectations

An issue that came up several times during the workshop, including in this discussion, centered on realistic expectations from introducing a new supermarket into a food desert, in terms of changes in food intake and ultimately BMI or other health outcomes. The natural experiments with which Cummins has been involved led him to realize, he said, that robust underlying theoretical models and the time frames in which we might realistically see effects are still not fully known. One successful outcome could simply be increasing the number of food stores available, but a secondary outcome would be to see changes in health behaviors and then impacts on obesity or the prevalence of diabetes. Changes in important health behaviors and outcomes may take longer to ascertain than most current funding mechanisms allow. Diez Roux suggested looking at proximal outcomes in the short term, rather than trying to detect more distal effects.

Cummins also suggested making more use of complementary activities, such as mailings to residents or incentives, and evaluating the effect of these initiatives combined with changes in supply.

One workshop participant questioned whether food desert health outcomes are really due to limited food access or perhaps more likely to limited healthcare access. Diez Roux agreed the issues are confounded because the real world is complex, and it is difficult to separate the causal effect of food access. Methodologically, researchers attempt to create boundaries through a variety of statistical controls. Cummins said spatial analytic approaches to measure access using GIS (geographic information systems) in longitudinal studies may help avoid the problem of using administrative boundaries, which may shift over time, as a proxy for neighborhoods. People have different perceptions of neighborhood boundaries. Using census tracts as a proxy, in his opinion, also has weaknesses that qualitative research reveals. Questions remain about what is the most relevant and comparable spatial environment. Diez Roux agreed that a census tract is not ideal, but may serve as a useful although imperfect proxy for the most relevant spatial context.

Community and Interdisciplinary Initiatives

Reedy summarized several questions from workshop participants related to work within communities. Partnering with community groups to conduct research is important in this kind of research, said Diez Roux, particularly in evaluating natural experiments and conducting qualitative studies.

Studies have looked at various community benefits of addressing food issues. Urban agriculture is promoted in some cities to increase local food production, as well as to increase physical activity. Other studies have looked at the effects of using local government subsidies to encourage the opening of retail outlets that carry healthy foods: for example, if housing prices increase as a result, the tax base grows and the public investment has a positive fiscal return. Similarly, in the United Kingdom, retail leverage generation (planning gain) is considered a tool to improve the local economy through providing employment and upgrading public facilities such as sidewalks and other infrastructure. Despite concerns about the impact of a large store on smaller Glasgow retailers, the same number of small stores were in business 18 months later in the area that Cummins studied.

To close the session, Diez Roux emphasized the need for interdisciplinary research among epidemiologists, geographers, economists, and urban planners. Reedy expressed agreement on behalf of the other panelists and workshop participants.

4

Diet and Health Evidence to Support Improved Food Access

The interventions to improve food deserts center on increasing the intake of healthy foods. Those healthy foods include whole grains, fruits and vegetables, fat-free rather than whole milk, and drinking fewer calorically sweetened beverages. The excess availability of energy-dense snacks and fast foods in food deserts is a concern because both have been linked to obesity, and current interventions have attempted to increase the availability of healthy foods to mitigate those effects in food deserts; thus, presentations in this session addressed the possible public health outcomes of increasing healthy food intake. The speakers in this session focused on evidence-based health consequences of these changes in terms of obesity, cancer, and cardiovascular diseases.

EFFECTS OF SELECTED DIETARY FACTORS ON OBESITY

Richard Mattes, of Purdue University, stated that an increase in the consumption of healthy foods will not necessarily reduce body weight. In fact, only the case of reducing caloric beverage intake showed consensus on the link between change in diet and weight loss. Culture and learned associations often govern what people prefer to eat. He counseled caution in making the best choices about the interventions to pursue if the goal is reducing obesity. In short, there are no easy fixes.

Healthy Food and Changes in Weight

Fruits and Vegetables

Mattes suggested that the message in the media to "load up" on fruits and vegetables as a way to lower weight is misleading without considering overall energy intake. The Nurses Health Study, for example, which tracked almost 75,000 people over a 12-year period, showed that greater fruit and vegetable intake led to lower weight gain in women but not reduced weight for participants or for their children (He et al., 2004). Greater fruit and vegetable consumption alone will not reduce weight without the qualification to moderate energy intake.

Whole Grains

The next food category that Mattes discussed was whole versus refined grains. The line of reasoning behind encouraging consumption of whole grains is that they are higher in fiber and increase satiety, and therefore, people will eat less. Data from the Nurses Health Study indicate that greater intake of whole grain products was associated with reduced weight gain but provided little or no benefit for weight loss compared to consumption of refined grain products over the course of the 12-year study period (Liu et al., 2003). Other recent studies, both short and longer term, have shown similar results.

Milk

Drinking reduced-fat versus whole milk does not benefit weight management. Higher-income people purchase more low-fat milk and lower-income people purchase more whole milk, even when prices are the same, according to the Continuing Survey of Food Intake by Individuals (CSFII). The prevailing belief is that weight improves by switching to lower-fat dairy products. However, the Growing Up Today study (Berkey et al., 2005) and the National Health and Nutrition Examination Survey (Beydoun et al., 2008) actually show an increase in body mass index among children who drink fat-free and low-fat milk. This may reflect reverse causality in that heavier individuals choose lower-fat products to manage their weight, but it cannot be concluded that simply including lower-fat dairy products in the diet or substituting them for higher-fat products will promote weight loss.

Sweetened Beverages

Whereas eating or drinking these healthier foods does not reduce weight, evidence is stronger that drinking caloric beverages has a detrimental effect. Consumption of sweetened beverages is now about 40 gallons per capita and has clearly gone up in concert with the rise in BMI and obesity in the population (see Figure 4-1). On average, Americans now get about 21 percent of their total energy intake from beverages, almost double the amount in 1965 (Duffey and Popkin, 2007).

Beverages of all types seem to increase energy intake. In a study in which participants consumed various foods in liquefied and whole form, total energy intake was higher over the course of a day with the beverage form. The consumption of energy-yielding beverages seems to lead to a lack of dietary compensation, positive energy balance, and weight gain, although he acknowledged some controversy about whether there are sufficient data to move forward in terms of policy. Data specific to soft drink consumption from the Nurses Health Study showed that the weight

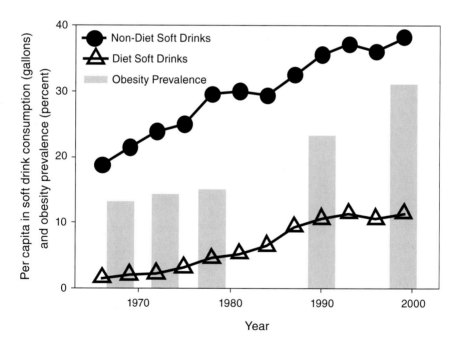

FIGURE 4-1 Soft drink consumption, 1970-2000.
SOURCE: USDA ERS, 2000. Reprinted with permission from Susan E. Swithers, Purdue University.

of individuals who drank nutritively sweetened beverages increased, while those who switched to nonnutritive "diet" drinks had a weight plateau (Schulze et al., 2004).

EFFECTS OF SELECTED DIETARY FACTORS ON CARDIOVASCULAR DISEASE AND CANCER

In contrast to obesity, research into the effects of diet on cardiovascular disease and cancer has shown a more positive link, said Frank Hu of Harvard University. Before discussing different categories of foods, he reviewed the hierarchy of evidence that nutrition researchers use in making clinical recommendations. The strength and consistency of evidence across different studies, biological plausibility, and responsive relationships are all needed to assess causal relationships between a food and a health outcome.

Fats and Carbohydrates

"Good" and "bad" fats have received much attention, with Americans encouraged to eat, for example, more healthy fats from plant-based oils and nuts rather than deep-fried food and stick margarine. The type of fat—the quality of the fats consumed, rather than total fat—has been shown to have a relationship to coronary heart disease (Hu et al., 1997) (see Figure 4-2). Fats have not generally increased breast cancer risk. There is fairly consistent evidence that higher consumption of red and processed meats is associated with increased risk of colorectal cancer, although it may not be due to the saturated fat in those products.

The study of carbohydrates has shifted from classification by their chemical structure to a focus on glycemic index and glycemic load. In this paradigm, the greater the amount of refined carbohydrates and sugar, the higher the glycemic load. He reported on research that found a strong positive association between a high glycemic load diet and the risk of coronary heart disease (CHD), especially among overweight and obese individuals who are more insulin resistant (Liu, 2000).

Plant-Based Foods

A systematic review of nuts, fruits, vegetables, and whole grains consistently showed that higher consumption of these foods is significantly associated with decreased risk of both coronary heart disease and stroke (Hu and Willett, 2002). They have not been associated with overall reduced cancer mortality, but have shown benefits for some individual types of cancers, including mouth, lung, and stomach cancers. The World

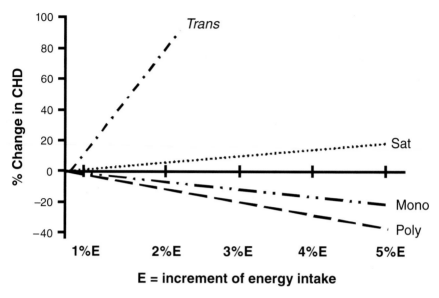

FIGURE 4-2 Effect of types of fat on coronary heart disease.
SOURCE: Hu et al., 1997.

Cancer Research Fund concluded that some non-starchy fruits and vegetables may protect against specific cancers.

Dairy Products

Hu characterized dairy as a "much more complicated story," with
potential benefits and potential problems. Although they are a good
source of many important nutrients, dairy products have also been associated with higher body weights among children and may increase risks
of some hormone-related cancers. He distinguished between fat-free and
whole milk. Replacing high-fat dairy with low-fat was associated with
lower risk of CHD and Type 2 diabetes.

Soft Drinks

Hu concurred with Mattes about the problems of soft drinks. In addition to weight gain, the Nurses Health Study and other research has
shown an association between soft drink consumption and the risk of
diabetes and CHD. Limited evidence from that study and several others
showed an association with pancreatic cancer, although those findings
were not unanimous.

The Bottom Line

Hu said the evidence is "pretty solid" that plant-based foods—including whole grains, fruits and vegetables, nuts, legumes, and healthy vegetable oils—are beneficial for cardiovascular disease (CVD) prevention. These foods are basically an indication of a high-quality diet. Diets high in saturated fat, trans fat, or refined sugars, including some starchy food, are detrimental for both diabetes and CVD. Sugar-sweetened beverages increase the risk of obesity, diabetes, and perhaps CVD.

The findings are less specific about the link between diet and cancer. The recommendation of the World Cancer Research Fund focuses on body weight and physical activity because these are more important than individual foods and nutrients in terms of cancer prevention.

DISCUSSION: HEALTH CONSEQUENCES

Wendy Johnson-Askew, of the National Institute of Diabetes and Digestive and Kidney Diseases at the National Institutes of Health (NIH), moderated the discussion on health consequences of healthy foods and, particularly among the less healthy options, sweetened beverages. Understanding the science can help guide the policy-making process, by either encouraging or discouraging the intake of specific foods.

Small Changes

Johnson-Askew launched the session by suggesting to Mattes that even the slightly reduced intake caused by eating more fiber, as reported in the Nurses Health Study, may have some significance in the long term. Mattes replied that small imbalances do add up over time, but not to as great an extent as reported in the popular media. Because the initial weight gain also increases the energy needed to sustain that weight, the original small positive energy balance does not continue to increase weight gain.

Along these lines, a participant noted that since the interest in weight stems from an interest in people's health, maybe separating the two does not move the conversation further. Any action, said Mattes, has positives and negatives. So a particular dietary intervention may cause weight gain at the same time that it reduces the risk for certain chronic diseases. The role of scientists is to provide policy makers with this information so that they can make evidence-based decisions.

Healthy Eating

One workshop participant suggested focusing on the Healthy Eating Index (HEI, developed by the U.S. Department of Agriculture), rather than BMI, as a proximal indicator of access to good food. Hu agreed that the revised HEI is a good measure of overall diet quality, and it is overall quality, rather than just individual nutrients, that contribute to our health. Mattes said from an obesity perspective, the time has come to abandon the idea that there is a single cause of obesity that a particular diet will correct. Just as it was once believed that a single treatment for cancer could be possible, it is now clear that obesity is caused by diet composition for some people, energy expenditure for others, and eating frequency or portion size for someone else. Mattes mentioned that more individualized interventions may be more appropriate for changing health outcomes. Another concern about more generalized recommendations is that some people have counterreactions to various changes: for example, about 15 percent of people with elevated cholesterol or blood pressure show an increase when they eat a fat-restricted or low-sodium diet, so this recommendation actually runs counter to this subgroup's good health. Hu agreed that there may be no silver bullet for curing obesity, and the data suggest that diet quality is more important than a specific type of low-fat or low-carbohydrate diet. Johnson-Askew noted that the issue of BMI as a marker of health is under debate by her and her colleagues at NIH.

Taxes and Subsidies

Should soda and other sugar-sweetened beverages be taxed? Mattes said the issue from an obesity perspective needs to be more about caloric beverages in general, not just soft drinks. Although sweetened soft drinks and fruit drinks are the largest source of refined carbohydrates and thus are a good target, the probability of a positive energy balance is likely to be as great from consuming milk, sports drinks, sugary gourmet teas and coffees, or fruit juice. The issue stems from the medium in which the energy is derived. Beverages, for reasons still unknown, seem to escape regulatory mechanisms. Mattes noted that people do not reduce their food intake when they consume beverages with calories.

Hu supported a soda tax for sweetened soft drinks, but not for diet soda, fruit juices, or other beverages for two reasons: (1) the evidence is more solid for sugar-sweetened beverages, and (2) these drinks are a clear and easily defined target.

Given the situation with food deserts and the prices of many healthy foods, one participant wondered about the fairness of promoting foods that not everyone can afford. Hu acknowledged that the prices of fruits and vegetables have increased, which perhaps should be addressed on a policy level. To make the consumption of healthier foods more affordable, government subsidies could be provided to specialty crops rather than to commodity crops such as corn. Employers perhaps could reward workers who follow a healthy diet and exercise regularly. Mattes said fairness is one reason he is not in favor of a soda tax, because it differentially isolates low-income populations, even though he recognizes the role of these beverages in the energy-balance problem.

Snacks and Extra Calories

Mattes said his review of the literature indicates that meal frequency, particularly snacking, may be a substantive contributor to weight gain. Americans are eating perhaps an extra half-meal or so per day, often a high-calorie snack. Hu said reducing soft drinks and unhealthy snacks are two main problems to address in improving health.

5

Ameliorating Food Desert Conditions

Most of the second day of the workshop focused on interventions to change food deserts. Some of these interventions were designed as research intervention trials and these were discussed in session 4. Session 5 addressed several promising, although less formally evaluated, programs and policies that are currently under way to improve the food environment. These interventions range from incentives for grocery stores and supermarkets to locate in underserved areas, to city-wide programs to encourage healthier eating, and extend to support for small, corner-type stores and neighborhood-based farmers markets.

RESEARCH INTERVENTIONS

Researchers have been evaluating different interventions to ameliorate food desert conditions. These include efforts aimed at changing the food environment in many different ways.

Overview of Efforts to Change the Food Environment

Joel Gittelsohn, of Johns Hopkins University, presented an overview of efforts to change the food environment and reminded the group that food outlets—including supermarkets, small food stores, restaurants, and school and worksite cafeterias—are all part of the larger community nutrition environment. Policy, environmental, and individual variables

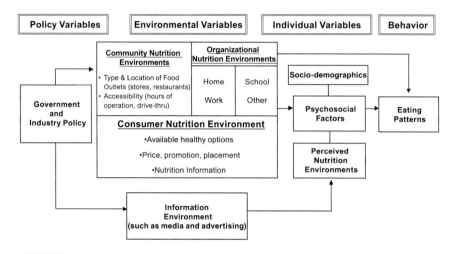

FIGURE 5-1 Model of community nutrition environments.
SOURCE: Glanz et al., 2005. Reprinted with permission from the *American Journal of Health Promotion.*

combine to affect eating patterns on an individual and collective basis (see Figure 5-1).

Given this caveat, changing the food environment has many potential benefits. Among these benefits, such changes can limit or expand the range of choices available to consumers, increase access to healthy foods, complement individual behavioral change programs, reach large numbers of people, and provide long-term sustainability if efforts are institutionalized. It is a practical way, perhaps the only practical way, to address the obesity epidemic. In addition to altering access, the food environment can also be changed within stores, within neighborhoods, and in other settings through provision of information and promotions to consumers. In all cases, the link between supply and demand is key to determining whether changes in the environment will be linked with healthier eating. As Gittelsohn termed it, the "trifecta" is to increase availability, reduce price, and promote healthier choices.

Availability in Large and Small Stores

Seymour et al. (2004) reviewed 11 supermarket intervention studies, 8 of which provided information about healthy foods to consumers and 3 of which combined information with changes in access, availability, and incentives. Six of the studies (four with information only) showed increases in sales of healthier foods, while five did not show a change. Of the three studies that also examined dietary data, one showed increased consumption of healthier foods and two did not register impacts. Based on this review, Gittelsohn concluded that informational shelf labeling seems to work, while incentives, in the form of coupons, had little impact. However, a longer duration of up to two years may be needed to show any significant change.

Since 2004-2005, researchers have conducted a number of intervention trials in small stores, which are often the main source of retail food purchases among low-income, ethnic, minority populations. Gittelsohn and a colleague are now in the process of reviewing 14 such studies: 5 studies confined to the stores and 9 that combined in-store interventions with community social marketing. These studies indicate a potential for success, as measured by reported improvements in fruit and vegetable sales, consumer psychosocial behaviors, healthy food purchasing patterns, and consumer diet. Challenges to increasing fruit and vegetable availability in small stores include convincing store owners to stock healthier foods, especially fresh fruits and vegetables that are perishable and require special handling. He suggested first trying to convince small store owners to stock less risky (e.g., nonperishable) healthy foods, such as low-sugar or high-fiber cereals. In many cases, store layouts pose a barrier; some are so enclosed that customers cannot touch a food item until they purchase it. These closed settings also severely limit social engagement between the customer and the clerk and therefore create barriers for nutrition education opportunities.

Price Manipulation

Types of price manipulation include lowering prices of healthy foods, offering coupons and other incentives, and increasing prices of unhealthy foods to subsidize lowering the costs of healthy foods. The CHIPS (Changing Individuals' Purchase of Snacks) study (French et al., 2001) showed that modifying the prices of low-fat snacks in vending machines increased sales and did not decrease profits. Other studies have looked at price subsidies in school cafeterias and showed that healthier food intake continued even when the subsidies stopped. Gittelsohn stated that research on price manipulation in stores as a public health intervention is needed, but one difficulty in setting up a price trial in a food store is that retailers are reluctant to share their pricing strategies or to give up control over this key aspect of their business.

Other questions to resolve in changing the food environment include how to build and sustain community support, the role of locally produced foods, and the optimal combination of institutions to involve. Certain aspects of the food environment have been commonly measured, while others still need examination. For example, sales of selected foods, such as fruits and vegetables, are commonly measured, while total sales, which represent total intake, are not; it is difficult to measure impacts without knowing the numerator and denominator. Psychosocial considerations that influence store manager decisions, which could affect their expectations for stocking healthy foods, are rarely measured. On the consumer side, the impact on behavior and on health, in terms of actual food preparation and diet and in terms of BMI, is rarely measured.

Studying the Introduction of a New Supermarket in a Food Desert

Neil Wrigley, of the University of Southampton, United Kingdom, reported on a "natural experiment" first mentioned on day 1 of the workshop: the opening of a new supermarket in a food desert—in this case, a supermarket regenerated in an urban underserved area of Leeds, England. In the late 1990s, he said, the metaphor of a "food desert" captured British policy makers' attention. Reports and inquiries linked trends in retail development in which food stores were moving outside of urban areas and toward the edge of town to the development of food deserts and to public health consequences. However, empirical evidence on key aspects of these linkages was limited.

The Leeds Urban Regeneration Supermarket Intervention Study (Wrigley et al., 2003) was set up to link the policy debate to an evidence base and to assess the impact of a non-healthcare intervention, specifically a retail provision intervention, on food consumption patterns. The study was developed rapidly in response to an opportunistic possibility to conduct a "natural experiment" when one of the UK's first urban regeneration partnership stores was being constructed. Although possibly overly ambitious, Wrigley said the study established important benchmarks for subsequent retail provision intervention studies and was characterized by high-quality social survey data collection.

The focus was Seacroft, an area of about 15,000 households in one of the most deprived wards of England. By the 1990s, it had a crumbling shopping center with poor levels of food retail provision. Buying food entailed either leaving the area or using a limited range of smaller stores. In partnership with the city, a labor union, and a government agency, a large Tesco supermarket plus 10 smaller shops and other facilities opened in 2000, amidst much fanfare including a visit from then-Prime Minister Tony Blair. The intent was to improve food access along with increasing employment and revitalizing the local economy.

The Leeds study involved a two-wave household panel survey: the first in summer 2000, five months before the supermarket opened, with 1,009 respondents; the second in summer 2001, seven months afterward, involving 615 of the original group. A separate repeatability survey and focus groups were also carried out. Of the respondents, 45 percent switched to using the new store as their main food source, and 31 percent (nearly three times more than before) reported that they walked to the store to food-shop rather than relying on vehicles (often either taxis or borrowed cars) to travel to places further away. Small but significant increases in fruit and vegetable consumption were found among users of the new store. Qualitative evidence from focus groups found that people appreciated the benefits relating to ease of access, affordability, quality, and safety, although some were worried about temptations to overspend and were concerned about more affluent shoppers coming from outside areas.

Wrigley reviewed the Leeds study, as well as the Glasgow study described by Steven Cummins (see Chapter 3), to draw conclusions about supermarket intervention studies. He recommended that future studies should take sample size-statistical power and endogeneity-simultaneity issues more seriously; attempt to assess unintended consequences of the intervention; try to separate the impacts of physical access, economic access, and choice on food consumption; and appreciate the linkages between existing intervention studies and the dynamics of the food environment. Natural experiments, he said, change reality. They do not take place in a scientific vacuum and can fundamentally change the public discourse. Retailers in the United Kingdom are sensitized to the issue of food deserts to further their "enlightened self-interest." There are now 35 urban regeneration partnership stores in the United Kingdom, and Tesco is opening up stores in south-central Los Angeles under its Fresh & Easy brand.

Wrigley concluded by noting that some academics in the United Kingdom are more comfortable with alternative food network solutions, rather than supermarkets, in addressing food deserts. While solutions such as farmers' markets have a role to play, he disagreed with his UK colleagues and questioned the extent to which they can penetrate socially excluded areas, at least in the United Kingdom, and have an impact on public health problems.

Working with Small Stores to Promote Healthy Eating

Guadalupe Ayala, of San Diego State University, described her research with *tiendas*, which she described as small Latino-Hispanic grocery stores with at least 50 percent of store shelf space devoted to food products, including fruits and vegetables, ready-to-eat foods, and meat. Also called *bodegas* by some Spanish speakers, these stores are very plentiful in Latino communities. They play important social and economic roles in both new and established immigrant-receiving communities, and for new immigrants they often serve as a gateway into U.S. communities. In studies funded by the USDA and the National Cancer Institute, Ayala found that households shop at these types of stores an average of eight times per month, and they represent 33 percent of a family's total food basket and 84 percent of a family's total produce purchases, with much of the rest purchased at supercenters.

Ayala said her research shows that working with tiendas and other small grocery stores may be an effective method to address the problem of food deserts. The study, Vida Sana Hoy y Mañana (Healthy Life Today and Tomorrow), examined the efficacy of a food marketing and environmental change intervention to promote sales and consumption of fruits and vegetables. Although Latinos eat more fruits and vegetables than other demographic groups, acculturation has a negative impact: the longer people have been in the United States, the lower is their fruit and vegetable intake (Duffey et al., 2008). The primary outcome measured in the study was the number of daily servings of fruits and vegetables. It secondarily measured their total variety, behavioral strategies to increase fiber, and psychosocial factors, such as perceived self-efficacy to purchase more produce.

The intervention was a randomized controlled trial in four North Carolina tiendas. It included employee and manager training, structural changes in the stores, and store-centered food marketing campaigns. The training enabled store personnel to become "fruit and vegetable specialists," as well as strengthen their selling and marketing strategies. The stores received $1,000 each to prepare and display packages of fruits and vegetables called "Pronto Paks." The food marketing campaign included recipes, point-of-purchase materials, and a radio program.

Consumer fruit and vegetable intake increased with this intervention by about one additional serving per day (see Figure 5-2). Self-efficacy in terms of purchasing and using fruits and vegetables declined, possibly because respondents felt less capable as more was learned and awareness heightened, especially in the short run.

Ayala noted some challenges in small-store interventions. The owners may be reluctant to participate in government programs. For example, researchers first suggested tapping into a program sponsored by the North Carolina Department of Agriculture to link food retail businesses with local farmers, but the tienda owners did not want to get involved. They have no mechanism for electronically tracking sales data, which makes it hard to know what is sold. Follow-up is especially difficult with new immigrant populations, with only about two-thirds located for follow-up 10 months after the intervention. Ayala said that in terms of identifying what foods to target in future interventions, Latino stores tend to stock far less low-fat dairy (and at higher relative prices) and more

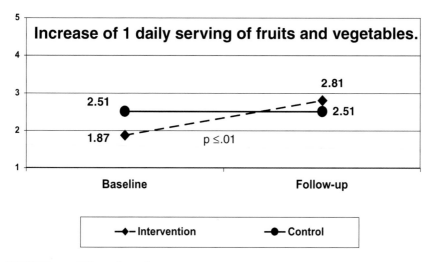

FIGURE 5-2 Effect of tienda intervention on consumption.
SOURCE: G. Ayala, 2009.

sugar-sweetened beverages and sweet and savory snacks, compared to non-Latino stores.

Farmers Markets in Low-Income Communities

Farmers markets, although a tiny percentage of the overall food environment, are expanding (see Box 5-1). Research from East Austin, Texas, shows some of the elements to consider in food deserts.

Andrew Smiley, of the Sustainable Food Center (SFC), discussed its experiences in establishing farmers markets in East Austin, Texas. A well-intentioned effort to establish a central market did not succeed in the long term. Instead, SFC has found that smaller markets near Women, Infants, and Children (WIC) clinics are meeting the community's needs.

A 1996 study of food access in East Austin found food desert conditions (SFC, 1995): two supermarkets, other retail food outlets with poor variety and generally higher prices, and transportation to outlets outside the neighborhood expensive and difficult to arrange. The targeted area is a predominantly minority low-income community, with about 25 percent of the 24,000 residents under age 12. Of the 38 convenience stores in the neighborhood, fewer than half stocked milk and only 5 stocked all of the ingredients for a well-balanced meal. One solution, still in operation, was a bus route, specifically designed to reach supermarkets, that has not been evaluated for its impact.

BOX 5-1
Farmers Markets: Small But Growing Market Segment

Farmers markets occupy a small, but growing share of the U.S. food environment. According to workshop participant Debra Tropp, of the USDA Agricultural Marketing Service, farmers markets accounted for about $1.2 billion in sales in 2007, up from $812 million in 2002, or a 30 percent increase after adjusting for inflation. In 2008, there were 4,685 markets operating, up from 1,755 in 1994, with more than 135,000 farms involved.

Consumers are also using farmers markets as a source of fresh fruits and vegetables. Workshop participant Heidi Blanck, of the Centers for Disease Control and Prevention (CDC), mentioned a recent consumer survey conducted by the CDC and the National Cancer Institute on the use of farm-to-consumer venues and food attitudes and behavior. The survey showed that in 2007, one in five adults self-identified as primary food shoppers reported shopping at farmers markets (20.1 percent). When asked how often in the summer they purchased fruits and vegetables from a farm-to-consumer venue (i.e., farmers market, farm stand, pick your own farm, community-supported agriculture), 56.1 percent of primary food shoppers reported at least monthly use and 27.1 percent reported weekly use. Weekly use was higher among middle-aged and older adults and lower in the South and Northeast compared to the West. Weekly use did not differ by sex, race or ethnicity, education, or income.

SOURCES: H. Blanck, 2009; D. Tropp, 2009; USDA NASS, 2009.

Another proposed solution was a centrally located farmers market. SFC already operated a large market in downtown Austin and several smaller ones at WIC clinics in other neighborhoods. To open a large market in East Austin's Saltillo Plaza in 2003, SFC recruited vendors, promoted the market, took out insurance, managed operations, and carried out a host of other tasks. Despite outreach, special events, and other efforts, evaluation indicated that the market lacked sufficient support for the resources expended. The majority of sales were due to WIC Farmers' Market Nutrition Program (FMNP) vouchers, but these went only to fruit and vegetable farmers. Surveys and focus groups indicated that word of mouth generated awareness about the market, but people felt it was inconvenient for regular shopping. Those who did come especially valued the fruits and vegetables and, across income levels, the idea of supporting local farmers. However, there just were not enough customers to justify SFC or farmers' costs, and SFC decided to close the market in 2005.

Produce sellers were still interested in additional sales outlets, and customers with FMNP vouchers still wanted to purchase their products.

In an alternative and still successful approach, SFC decided to support very small (one or two) farmers markets located next to WIC clinics. WIC clinic markets are not as staff-intensive, and WIC staff members are good partners in outreach. Six of these clinics are now operating.

Discussion: Research Interventions

Terry Huang, of the National Institute of Child Health and Human Development at NIH, moderated the session on food desert intervention research. Main points included the need for multicomponent interventions, formative research, and more robust price manipulation trials.

Making Farmers Markets Viable

Huang related questions about setting up farmers markets, especially near WIC clinics. Smiley said that the state FMNP program made it easier for individual clinics to participate. SFC has liability insurance for the markets it coordinates, which greatly eased liability concerns. Some neighborhood convenience stores saw the markets as a threat. This required some outreach to explain that the small markets take FMNP vouchers almost exclusively and did not pose any competition. In answer to a question about locating markets so that they simultaneously straddle more and less affluent neighborhoods, Smiley noted that determining new sites is both a physical and a psychological issue. In the case of Austin, for example, location vis-à-vis a highway that runs through the city makes a big difference psychologically and logistically.

Incentives

Gittelsohn noted that incentives can go to shoppers or to store owners. In addition to coupons, he has been involved with trials in which, for example, a shopper gets one free (healthy) item for every four purchased. However, these have not been successful in small stores, in part because owners worry about consumers abusing the incentives. Ayala said she was involved in an experiment in which a customer would get one free pound of produce for every 10 pounds purchased. It became too much of a burden for the store owners and was not sustainable.

In contrast, incentives to small-store owners, such as $25-50 gift cards they can use with wholesalers, have been promising, Gittelsohn said. Ayala said interviews with tienda owners in California revealed that they try to make every square foot of the store as profitable as possible. They are willing to try something for a month to see if it will bring in more customers or profit.

The cost for small stores to equip themselves to sell fresh produce varies. In California, store owners told Ayala it would cost between $5,000 and $10,000 for refrigeration units to stock fruits and vegetables. However, even with small additions that cost $1,500 to set up, changes were seen in customers' dietary intake. In addition, states and counties may have different policies and regulations, which have an impact on implementation costs for store owners. Defraying theses costs would help store owners that usually operate on thin profit margins.

The Role of Price

As noted throughout the workshop, price matters. Gittelsohn said literature is scarce on food store price manipulations for public health interventions, making it difficult to arrive at definitive conclusions about what does and does not work. That is, although it is widely known that lowering price is used to increase sales volume, there is little documentation or evaluation of the use of prices to improve the healthfulness of diets. Intuitively, increased availability and point-of-purchase promotion encourage people to try new foods, but they have to cost less or at least about the same price as less healthy alternatives. Wrigley observed that improved access and improved price frequently go together, so it is hard to distinguish one from the other. He suggested that urban regeneration stores could perhaps carry out pricing experiments. Smiley noted that testing perceptions is important, too. For example, a survey found some people do not shop at farmers markets because they perceive them to be more expensive, even when prices are comparable.

Ayala said that low-fat milk is consistently more expensive than whole milk across Latino stores, which is not the case in other communities. Latino households drink more whole milk, and the price differential may be because of market demand. Another factor that may discourage sales of lower-fat products relates to packaging: low-fat products sometimes do not have "Vitamin D" on their labels. While there are many barriers to changing learned behaviors and preferences, the price difference would have to be resolved first before educational campaigns are considered.

Popkin noted that food processors continually manipulate price as part of their business practices. For example, food processors have found prepackaged vegetable servings to be successful, but these items are also priced well and highly promoted, which makes the separate elements difficult to evaluate. Wrigley reiterated findings from focus groups about worries from exposure to the temptations of full-scale retailers. The issue of being tempted to overspend fixed budgets is a big issue, and obviously a price-related issue.

Multicomponent Approaches

Multi-institutional, multicomponent approaches are a natural extension of current research looking at single parts of the food environment. Formative research that involves community participatory processes would help plan interventions. The type of foods to focus on may vary by location and culture, but sweetened beverages seem to be a key problem across many low-income settings. Huang asked whether beverages should be addressed from both the demand and the supply sides: discouraging their purchase but also working with companies to reformulate the product. Gittelsohn has done some preliminary work with local manufacturers and distributors in terms of changing the mix offered to stores. Customers claim they do not eat healthy foods because the foods are not available, cost too much, or are of poor quality; on the other hand, store owners claim they do not stock the healthy foods because nobody buys them. Almost as a mediator, public health and other specialists can concurrently convince store owners to increase supply and work with consumers to increase demand.

Another need, according to Ayala, is to better enumerate stock inventory. The type and number of products in tiendas is far different than those in convenience stores, and Ayala asserts that food desert conditions may not exist in predominantly Latino Hispanic communities. It would be interesting to understand whether the food environment is one of the factors that explain the "Hispanic paradox," which suggests that first-generation Latinos have better health outcomes than their acculturated counterparts despite greater poverty and lower socioeconomic status.

E-commerce

The question was raised about using the telephone or Internet to place orders to lower costs and increase access. Smiley said the SFC operates a Farm-to-Work program, a subscription program for employees at partner work sites. In another project in Austin, WIC families pre-order their full mix of groceries for delivery to centralized locations. Gittelsohn said cell phones are so widespread that using them in this way could offer an interesting possibility. Wrigley said the origins of e-commerce in the United Kingdom were to reach underserved markets. An experiment in Newcastle from 1980 to 1982 involved computer access from public libraries in underserved areas of the city to place grocery orders. Ayala observed that the digital divide is not as pronounced as it was a few years ago, but interpersonal relationships are too strong to make e-commerce for food a viable option, at least in the Latino community. Diez Roux warned about creating new problems while supposedly fixing others. For example, having a store or other destination to travel to promotes physical activity and social interactions. The much bigger problem is the way in which environments affect a variety of health behaviors at the same time.

Huang asked workshop attendees for further observations. Sarah Trehaft, of PolicyLink, urged listening to community voices in discussing food desert measurements, policies, and interventions. Popkin agreed that community participation and feedback are essential to successful approaches and outcomes.

POLICY INTERVENTIONS

Research interventions to modify the food environment are attractive because they are fundable and measurable, however, research interventions are merely one solution to solving food deserts in communities. The policies and programs discussed by the next session also aimed at improving access to healthy food in food deserts through supermarkets, corner stores, farmers markets, and other outlets. While these interventions were not set up as research experiments, they are, nevertheless, an interesting mix of initiatives launched by government agencies and grassroots efforts that began at the community level and became more widespread (see Box 5-2). Most have or are planning some types of formative research and evaluation.

Determining Sites for New Supermarkets

In developing strategies to increase the number of supermarkets in food deserts, it is important to understand the prevailing business model of U.S. supermarket chains. According to William Drake, a former supermarket executive now with Cornell University, most food retailers are aware of the issues of food security and urban food deserts. However, a combination of internal capabilities, external trade area characteristics, economic realities, and intolerance for risk raises difficult barriers to overcome and hence the difficulty for supermarkets to site new stores in food deserts.

Drake described the prototype for most supermarkets in the United States today: large (48,000 square feet), with plentiful parking (250 spaces), and sales volume of $400,000 per week, all difficult to achieve in most core urban areas. About two-thirds of the nation's 34,000 supermarkets belong to a chain, defined as stores with at least 11 units. The profit margin is thin, in the range of 1.5 to 1.75 percent of sales. To maximize profit, the most successful chains are "finely tuned machines" that know their target consumers and operate in ways to attract them to buy. To diverge from their model, he said, is very inefficient and more likely to fail. Supermarkets in the past 20 years have tended to locate in middle- and upper-

---

BOX 5-2
Top-Down and Bottom-Up Approaches

Top-down and bottom-up approaches have been used to launch and coordinate efforts to improve food access. "Top down" refers to initiatives emanating from a government agency or other institution; "bottom up" refers to initiatives that begin in neighborhoods or in community-based organizations and become larger programs or policies.

For example, in 2002 the New York City Department of Health initiated a concerted effort to focus health intervention in the South Bronx, Central and South Brooklyn, and East and Central Harlem. These were areas with high rates of poor health outcomes, including obesity and diabetes. Survey data also show that these areas have the lowest rates of fruit and vegetable consumption in the city. These District Public Health Offices have been the central point for four food access projects: (1) improving food choices in corner stores, (2) increasing the number of farmers markets, (3) increasing or at least maintaining the number of supermarkets, and (4) encouraging fruit and vegetable vendors. Although involving the community, these initiatives began at "the top."

In Philadelphia in 1992, the nonprofit Food Trust began a community-level mission to "ensure that everyone has access to affordable, nutritious food." The organization helped set up farmers' markets in low-income neighborhoods to improve access to affordable nutritious food and now manages 30 markets in the greater Philadelphia area.

---

income suburban locations where they have a good chance of meeting their targets. Chains also tend to site new stores relatively close to their existing outlets for a number of economic and logistic advantages.

Once a general geographic area is identified, the chain makes site-specific decisions. Its business analyses rely on variables such as projected sales, occupancy costs, and labor expenses, among others. These models work less well in urban settings because the underlying data are often underestimated or misrepresented. For example, it is difficult to gauge sales when the current competitors are small corner stores rather than other supermarkets. Without good knowledge of an area, Drake said, siting decisions are more prone to fail.

State and local governments can assist retailers in entering urban markets by providing real estate or establishing public transportation stops to commercial locations and food stores, particularly in inner cities. Yet the fact remains that locations in urban food deserts do not fit the positioning strategy of most large chain supermarket operations. As an alternative, he suggested working with voluntary and cooperative food wholesalers, the segment of the industry that serves independent retailers. Independent retailers are better able to customize a positioning strategy and adapt to local conditions than the larger chains. Another idea is to target specific retail stores that have a business model with a better chance of success in urban inner-city markets. Known as limited assortment hard discounters, these stores offer healthy foods at competitive prices but with a more limited assortment.

Policies to Encourage Supermarket Entry

As reported by Drake, the average supermarket in the United States is about 48,000 square feet and is set in a suburban location with plentiful parking. However, several presenters reported on variations that fit better in urban environments: smaller stores, perhaps 12,000 to 15,000 square feet, with more limited parking and convenient public transport or shuttles to help shoppers take their food home.

John Weidman, of the Philadelphia-based the Food Trust, described how the nonprofit built on its many years of community food work to help develop the Fresh Food Marketing Initiative in Pennsylvania. As in Chicago, New York City, and other places, mapping in Philadelphia showed the coincidence of a lack of supermarkets with a high incidence of diet-related diseases. The mapping study sparked the interest of the City Council, which requested that the Food Trust convene a group of public health, economic development, government, and supermarket industry representatives to understand why stores did not locate in these communities and what policies could fix the problem. The State of Pennsylvania also held hearings, and in 2004, this work culminated in the Fresh Food Financing Initiative (FFFI), the nation's first public–private funding initiative set aside for retailers to open and update stores in underserved food deserts.

The FFFI is a $120 million initiative that funds food retail projects in underserved areas. It provides grants of up to $250,000 per store and loans of up to $2.5 million per store. Since 2004, it has funded 58 stores of various sizes that have provided almost 3,500 jobs. Most of the larger stores are independent or small, locally based chains. Spatial analysis confirms that these stores have gone into many areas with the greatest need. The Food Trust is now working on evaluating the health outcomes and expanding its efforts in other states, including New York, Louisiana, Illinois, and New Jersey.

Cathy Nonas, of New York City's Department of Health & Mental Hygiene, described how the city is trying to increase, or at least maintain, the number of supermarkets operating in high-need neighborhoods. A city planning standard was set to aim for a store of 15,000 square feet to serve on average 10,000 people living in a five-block radius. A supermarket commission was established, with assistance from the Food Trust, to look at zoning regulations and tax incentives. Some city-owned spaces have been identified as potential sites for new stores. At the same time, community-based organizations and unions are working with city and state officials to stop the closing of supermarkets, and they have had some success in Harlem.

SMALL STORES

A point brought up throughout the workshop is that improving the food offerings of existing stores in a community can be a feasible solution to accomplish the goal of making healthy foods convenient and affordable. For example, on the first day of the workshop, Joseph Sharkey suggested focusing on where people currently shop when he presented an overview of the rural Brazos Valley. Gittelsohn reported that research into small-store interventions has greatly increased since 2004, and Ayala shared her findings from small stores in Latino communities. In this session, Nonas and Weidman explained several small-store programs in New York and Philadelphia.

Healthy Bodegas in New York City

The New York City Department of Health & Mental Hygiene has targeted areas in three parts of the city where it is trying to improve food access, as previously reported in Box 5-2. Nonas explained that through the Healthy Bodega Initiative, the department is encouraging existing stores in these areas to improve their offerings of healthy foods. In a first phase, three district public health officers worked with about 350 bodegas each (more than 1,000 total) to increase availability and purchases of low-fat milk. Extensive consumer education accompanied outreach to the bodegas (Figure 5-3). In the next phase targeting fruits and vegetables, more than 450 bodegas participated; the smaller number was chosen based on the store's interest in selling and increasing its quantity of fresh produce. Depending on the store's characteristics, the department helped bodega owners increase quantity, improve quality, provide prepackaged items, market healthy foods better, or obtain the appropriate permits to sell processed produce and produce in front of the store or on the stoop.

The two campaign phases saw large increases in sales of low-fat milk and fruits and vegetables, although Nonas acknowledged that it is hard to evaluate the effect apart from other factors, such as offering WIC participants coupons for low-fat milk. She listed challenges in sustaining the initiative: not enough staff to reach out to so many stores and visit them sufficiently, the need to balance outreach efforts between community

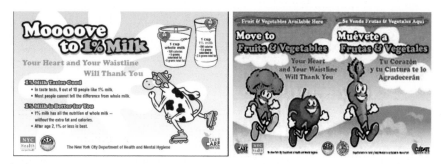

FIGURE 5-3 Consumer materials used in the Healthy Bodega Initiative.
SOURCE: C. Nonas, 2009.

buy-in and bodegas, limited infrastructure in many bodegas (such as refrigeration and storage), haphazard distribution systems, and the need for micro-loans and education to make the necessary improvements.

The department is now working more closely with fewer bodegas to make more sustainable and substantive changes and to increase healthy food options in those stores. Each district public health officer works with 20 bodegas, chosen to ensure that each resident is within walking distance of at least one healthier bodega, which they can visit at least twice a month. As Nonas said, if three bodegas are located on a block, maybe only one needs to carry fruits and vegetables. Nonas noted that the department also works with these stores to decrease tobacco ads and identify healthier items in the store with promotional materials, and works with other city agencies and organizations (such as milk distributors, produce distribution sites, micro-loaners, and permitting centers) to make it easier for city bodegas to stock and sell healthier items.

Making Healthy Food at Corner Stores Kid Friendly

John Weidman reported that the Food Trust works with Philadelphia corner stores where children stop for snacks. After starting a school nutrition program, the Food Trust did research on the role of corner stores in children's nutritional status. They found that children consumed about 600 calories in snacks, almost all of them unhealthy, spending about $2 per day. In a pilot program in five stores in North Philadelphia, refrigerated coolers were set up with fresh fruit. The attention-grabbing coolers and attractive packages appealed to kids, and sales were brisk. A private operator has taken on and expanded distribution to 50 stores, which solves the problem of a sustainable distribution network. A plan to create kid-pleasing water bottles is next.

Initial evaluations show kids purchasing items with less fat and fewer calories. The owners are purchasing more healthy items, and the children's knowledge of healthy eating is improving. The Food Trust is currently midway through a more rigorous randomized study to track a group of children for three years and look at BMI and calorie reduction.

FARMERS MARKETS AND OTHER ALTERNATIVES IN LOW-INCOME COMMUNITIES

As described above, farmers markets are a small but growing part of the food environment in the United States. Across income levels, consumers have shown they are willing to frequent these markets and, in many cases, they prefer the social interaction and direct contact with the growers. At the same time, as Smiley described, they need to be convenient and worthwhile from the point of view of both the buyer and the seller. Panelists shared their experiences from markets in several cities, as well as more cross-cutting lessons about community buy-in and the vital connection with government programs.

Health Bucks for Fresh Fruits and Vegetables

Nonas described how the New York City Department of Health & Mental Hygiene has looked for ways to support low-income residents in purchasing fresh produce at farmers markets, in part by increasing the number of farmers markets in the target areas and enabling them to accept Electronic Benefit Transfers (EBT) from participants in the USDA's Supplemental Nutrition Assistance Program (SNAP, formerly know as the Food Stamp Program).

As an incentive to shop at neighborhood farmers markets, the city distributes "Health Bucks," which are $2 coupons for the purchase of fresh fruits and vegetables. In 2005, the program began by distributing these coupons to community-based organizations for their constituents. The original program was so successful that in 2007, additional Health Bucks were distributed in the form of a $2 bonus for every $5 spent using EBTs at a farmers market. In addition, the department encouraged farmers to sell different types of healthy produce (such as peaches and plantains), and sales have been good. Health Bucks have been a major source of income for farmers selling at these markets and have ensured that markets profit in these low-income areas. Nonas mentioned that EBT sales have also skyrocketed since their introduction.

Nonas said it takes a multiagency effort to make Health Bucks successful and, more generally, to keep farmers markets in low-income communities thriving. An ongoing challenge is how to pay for EBT machines at the markets, as well as a market manager to oversee the machine and coordinate reimbursement to farmers. Also, she noted the need to continue access to fruits and vegetables when the farmers market season is over because most markets in these areas are not year-round.

Lessons from Philadelphia

The Food Trust's work with farmers markets has been successful in neighborhoods at all income levels, mentioned Weidman. In annual surveys, customers report significant vegetable intake and more frequent snacking with fruits and vegetables. He identified key components in making farmers markets successful in low-income communities:

- Strong management
- Site selection to locate a market in a place that works for the community and the vendors
- Strong community partnerships
- Connections with government programs
- Marketing

A pilot program in which each vendor stand had its own EBT machine resulted in increased usage. The machines processed credit cards too, so the farmers and other shoppers also benefited. Weidman suggested that this is maybe the future of vendor transactions as the economy becomes more "electronic."

Involving Communities in California

Andrew Fisher, of the Food Security Coalition, described the 250-member coalition as the connective tissue between advocacy and technical assistance. He discussed three projects in greater Los Angeles to provide insights about the role of the community in food desert projects: the Villa Parke Center Farmers' Market in Pasadena, Market-to-School project in Santa Monica, and urban agriculture project in Watts.

The Villa Parke Center Farmers' Market has operated in a low-income part of Pasadena for more than two decades. A benefit of this and other successful markets is that they build social capital as people interact with vendors and each other more so than in a supermarket. Many farmers hire helpers from within the community. Accepting government subsidy benefits is important to success in low-income communities: For this particular market, farmers agree to participate so they can also sell at a more lucrative market in downtown Pasadena.

Price is an issue at farmers markets in low-income communities for both shoppers and farmers. Shoppers are price-sensitive, but farmers also need to see a return on their labor. Product mix is crucial. Language and culture can create barriers between vendors and shoppers and affect sales, which is one reason that a community-organizing approach and local hiring are important.

The market-to-school project in Santa Monica also succeeded through community support. Although Santa Monica is generally a well-off community with no food deserts, Fisher noted that a large percentage of the school population is low income. The project began in 1997 when a parent worked with a local farmers market to improve the offerings of his child's cafeteria salad bar. It has since spread to all the schools in the district, and one-third of children now regularly eat salad for lunch. The project was successful because it had the support of the school district and food service personnel. The logistics have been time-consuming but not insurmountable.

Less successful, but a valuable lesson nonetheless in terms of the role of community support, was an urban agriculture project to provide vegetable gardens on a 2-acre plot near a housing project in Watts. The goal was to provide low- to no-cost healthy foods that could be grown year-round in the temperate Los Angeles climate and foster community interaction. Fisher said the project did not succeed because it was too top-down. The plan was presented to gardeners, some of whom were already tending plots, rather than involving them in planning how it would work. The gardeners were supposed to grow tomatoes and carrots when they knew growing herbs was more lucrative. In addition to poor design, friction between the staff and the gardeners worsened the situation.

Fisher noted that planners often see food as a private good, rather than a public benefit, or if so, under the purview of the federal government. As he commented, "There are no [local] departments of food in the country." Some policy solutions that could increase access on a community level include transportation changes, such as buses or shuttles, or a ban on lease restrictions that prevent new supermarkets from replacing those that close down. Public–private councils, now operating in about 100 communities around the country, also bring diverse stakeholders to the table to find ways to enhance food access.

Tapping into Public Funding

The benefits provided through SNAP and WIC, as well as Supplemental Security Income (SSI) and other federal and state assistance programs, are critical elements in making farmers markets a going concern in low-income communities.

August Schumacher, Jr., a former USDA undersecretary of farm and foreign agriculture services and now consultant with the Kellogg Foundation, elaborated on how changes in the SNAP and WIC Programs could further reduce rural and urban food deserts. SNAP retailers (such as corner stores and farmers markets) do not have to represent the bleak picture described in Detroit by Mari Gallagher (see Chapter 2).

Federal and state nutrition funding is evolving. Starting in 2009, more than 6 million WIC mothers and children nationwide will receive vouchers to buy fruits and vegetables in supermarkets and farmers markets. WIC mothers will receive $8 per month, and WIC-eligible children will receive $5 per month for fruit and vegetable purchases. He expressed hope that the amount increases. Schumacher noted that Congress will be reauthorizing the vital Child Nutrition legislation later in 2009 and 2010. He believes that increasing the provisions for healthy food purchases in this legislation—particularly, increasing the monthly funding for WIC mothers and children to purchase fruits and vegetables—would be exceptionally helpful in partially alleviating the growing incidence of obesity and diabetes among America's vulnerable children, many who live in food deserts.

Schumacher also reviewed the status of new funding to promote healthy food incentives in the 2008 Farm Bill. The provision within Section 4141 is for a $20 million pilot program under SNAP to explore how the immense program can improve the dietary and health status of eligible households. Regulations are being developed within USDA to set up pilot programs.

To support these evolving federal nutrition improvement programs, Schumacher cited a combination of foundations, states, and cities that fund healthy food incentives—such as those in Holyoke and Boston, Massachusetts, and San Diego, California—that allow SNAP, WIC, and SSI clients to receive "double vouchers" to increase their purchases of fruits and vegetables using SNAP EBT cards or WIC vouchers. He also noted that EBT cards could be an effective way to track fruit and vegetable purchases. Foundations such as the Wholesome Wave Foundation and the Humpty Dumpty Foundation provided funds in four states (California, Massachusetts, New York, and Connecticut) in 2008 and, with additional foundation partnerships, are considering expansion to eight more states in 2009.

Schumacher said the diversity of the American food system, in terms of farmers and shoppers, will lead to growth in the sector. Data from the USDA's Agricultural Census (USDA NASS, 2009) indicated 100,000 new farmers in the United States, with strong growth of Hispanic, Asian, Native American, and African-American farm operators. He is also optimistic about new demand drivers for fruits and vegetables, including an emphasis on child nutrition, healthier lunches and breakfasts at school, and expansion of SNAP and WIC use. He urged that new WIC vouchers add roadside stands to their permitted retail stores because many WIC mothers live in rural areas where farmers markets and full-service supermarkets are less prevalent. In addition, Schumacher suggested that funding for the Section 4141 Healthy Food Incentive program increase from $20 million to $100 million. He also said making it easier for farmers markets to get waivers to accept federal benefits would help them expand in low-income areas.

DISCUSSION: POLICY INTERVENTIONS

Robin McKinnon, of the National Cancer Institute at NIH, served as moderator for this panel discussion. The need for a connection between communities and food outlets ran through the questions and comments.

Supermarket Incentives

Drake said incentives at the state and local levels are especially important, such as helping to assemble real estate, job assistance, and training. Stores are only as good as their employees, and preventing turnover, which can be in excess of 100 percent per year in some inner-city stores, is a huge task. Transportation for shoppers and employees helps. Weidman suggested a federal-level equivalent to the FFFI for public–private funding initiatives.

Farmers Markets

One workshop participant expressed concern about a relationship between farmers markets and gentrification. Weidman said this has not occurred in Philadelphia, but rather there is a revitalization factor that benefits the community. Schumacher said that sellers or employees from within the community help make markets successful. Fisher noted that certified farmers market in California must work with the community. Successful markets take about a year to get organized, including a process of amassing community support.

The cost of setting up a farmers market varies. The Food Trust operates a network of markets, which helps consolidate the workload. Nonas pointed out that it makes a difference whether the market accepts EBT, which adds costs. Often middle-sized farmers have the hardest time dedicating the resources to sell at markets, and they need to make enough money for this to be worthwhile. Weidman said that there was some concern about whether the Philadelphia area had enough farmers to set up at all the markets. He said recent experience has shown there are plenty, including many younger farmers under the age of 30, an encouraging sign for the future of farming.

Community Outreach

As noted above, community acceptance is important to the success of farmers markets. Instilling ownership and buy-in is also important with supermarkets. Fisher said joint ventures have been helpful, such as a Pathmark in Newark, New Jersey, that partnered with the nonprofit New Community Corporation. Weidman noted that the bigger chains have not participated much in the FFFI, for reasons explained by Drake and others, but smaller independents have. Those that pay attention to community needs find it pays off. He cited the example of the Brown Family Shoprite, which heeded community requests to offer halal meats, now a best-selling item.

McKinnon asked about farmers markets in more dispersed rural areas. Schumacher said markets have been growing in rural areas, as he has seen in his work in Alabama and Mississippi. Weidman said that rural counties have also accessed the FFFI program.

6

Research Gaps and Needs

As described throughout the two days of the workshop, the purpose of food desert research is to understand factors that contribute to food deserts and ultimately to identify ways that facilitate change for health and non-health benefits. This is an emerging field that brings together a variety of disciplines, including public health, nutrition, economics, geography, and urban planning. The final session of the workshop summarized how additional research is essential for clarifying the causal link between the food environment and health and for informing researchers when they develop the most promising interventions. The study of food deserts and determining their impact on public health is extremely complex and requires multidisciplinary research approaches.

An overriding message of the workshop was that evidence shows food deserts exist in the United States along income, ethnic, and racial lines, both in urban and in rural areas. There are rich data on the local level and more general information on the national level, but it is yet to be determined if these findings from one area can be broadly applicable to areas with similar demographics.

The food environment is dynamic. New players are taking a growing percentage of the consumer's food dollar; these include supercenters, in particular, as well as farmers markets, dollar stores, convenience stores, and other outlets. Focusing only on supermarkets and grocery stores ignores the places where millions of Americans purchase some or all of their food.

Below are topics that were raised during the panels and summarized in this final wrap-up session.

DEVELOPMENT OF METHODOLOGY AND TOOLS

"Food access" was defined by presenters in various ways. A standard definition could help in making appropriate comparisons and furthering insight. One challenge is to resolve how the definition should incorporate such factors as geography, economics, and choice. If food access is determined using a spatial scale, the definition of "neighborhood" would benefit from further clarity and refinement.

Researchers reported on complementary instruments to measure food availability and affordability, including GIS, market basket surveys, other survey instruments, census data, and the Consumer Price Index. There is a strong desire (1) to develop and/or refine rigorous measures that are sensitive to the needs of diverse populations, and (2) to incorporate qualitative methods into research, in order to provide better information about issues such as consumer perceptions of food access.

Currently available data about food outlets from both public and private sources lack validation. Several presenters uncovered errors within national databases (such as those from Dun & Bradstreet and infoUSA) when they validated the measurement of these spatial data sets against actual visual measurements in specific neighborhoods, but it is unknown whether errors are random or somehow skewed to bias results. In addition, new census data, when available, will need to be used to investigate whether changes in the number of food outlets reflect population shifts. As noted above, the generalizability of local studies needs to be known before interventions can be applied on a broad scale.

Epidemiological Methods Combined with Multidisciplinary Approaches

Qualitative methods are also important for understanding the nuanced interaction between personal preferences and perceived access to quality food, which can then be compared to what is actually available. Challenges to understanding the links between food and health remain; they may best be met with multiple types of evidence from rigorous observational studies, natural experiments, simulations, and evaluations of evidence-based actions. Methods and tools from geography, demography, economics, psychology, sociology, urban planning, and policy can all help inform epidemiological research.

Longitudinal Studies

To date, most studies have been cross-sectional in that they compare different areas with different food environments. Longitudinal studies are crucial because they provide valuable information as the research follows the same population over time. Natural experiments can provide good information, but it is important that the experiments are theory driven and nuanced by population and other variables. Longer time frames are often critical for judging the effect of different interventions and possibly linking a population's food environment to its health. For natural experiments and other interventions, better surveillance methods can help researchers track information to see how an area is changing over time.

Policy and Program Evaluation

Policy and program interventions—such as those described in session five of the workshop (see Chapter 5)—were not generally set up by researchers. However, these activities may provide important opportunities for evaluation. To learn from both the successful and the unsuccessful elements, researchers could set up benchmarks for performance, sampling strategies, pre-testing of instruments, measurement of impacts on different sociodemographic groups, and process evaluations during interventions.

APPROACHES TO MEASURING FOOD DESERTS AND OUTCOMES

A theme that ran throughout the workshop was recognition of the complex physical and social environments in which food deserts are located. Approaches to understand some of the barriers can come from different disciplines working together.

Epidemiological

The causal links between food deserts and health have not been firmly established. Researchers may need to look at more proximal behavior changes, such as shopping behavior, and then look at dietary behavior and ultimately disease outcomes and weight. Understanding the link between food availability and changes in obesity requires a better understanding of these intermediate steps, particularly the effect on dietary intake and shopping and eating behaviors.

Research shows that people do not adjust caloric intake when they consume calories via beverages. It is not understood why this is so, nor are the implications clear for dietary recommendations. Randomized controlled trials on the effects of low-fat versus whole milk could be conducted, especially because children over age 2 and adults are currently advised to drink lower-fat milk.

Individual foods, overall diet quality, dietary patterns, and meal size and frequency play different roles in health outcomes. Because it is important to select the right interventions on which to focus resources, it makes sense to understand better which ones make the most difference.

Geospatial and Demographic

Although researchers aggregate and analyze data by geography, people may define their neighborhoods differently, in both urban and rural settings, which makes a difference in how they define food access. Their definitions may or may not coincide with administrative boundaries, census tracts, or other top-down categories. A better understanding of spatial behavior moves from merely the supply of stores, or of food within stores, to how people make decisions based on the spatial features around them. In addition, research to date has used the home as the central point, yet some people shop after work or in combination with other places they frequent during their day.

Formative research, with participation by community members, can help explore what stores can reasonably offer as healthier options that satisfy the preferences of consumers from diverse cultures. An example is the food dynamic in Latino communities, in terms of whether tiendas mitigate against food deserts more than small stores in other communities, as well as the relatively high use of whole milk.

Different issues across the lifespan came to light during the workshop. These issues include:

- the connection between food deserts and child BMI;
- teenagers' sensitivity to price, marketing messages, and eating patterns that fit their schedules;
- parents' purchasing decisions for themselves and their families; and
- aging adults with limited mobility, especially in areas without public transport.

Economic

The presentations underscored consumers' responsiveness to price. Additional research is necessary to gauge the impact of changing the prices of healthy and less healthy foods, as well as how purchasing behaviors vary by income, age, racial, and ethnic group. Will there be improved food and beverage choices if we increase the prices of caloric beverages, whole milk, or other unhealthy food choices or conversely reduce the prices of water, diet beverages, and low-fat milk? Research on price manipulation within stores as a public health intervention is limited, in part because of stores' reluctance to share pricing data. Urban regeneration stores in the UK may be more willing partners in this research than other commercial enterprises.

In addition, many argue that it is important to evaluate how individuals' perceptions affect their food access. People may have physical access, but not perceive they have economic access to healthy food.

Endogeneity is another issue that could benefit from further exploration. An endogenous factor or variable is one whose outcome is predicted by many of the same factors that arise within the model being studied. There are usually many unmeasured factors that affect both the endogenous factors and the outcome. For instance, access is endogenous to food deserts and health outcomes: those with access to supermarkets may have better diets because they choose to live near supermarkets, as healthy eating and nutrition are part of the decision-making for where residents locate. Alternatively, another endogenous factor might be the existence of a genetic susceptibility that enhances the taste of fat, increasing intake of fried fast foods and also affecting weight gain. Endogeneity may explain a great deal of the cross-sectional associations between measures of the food environment inside food deserts and food choices, obesity, and other health outcomes.

As presented at the workshop, small stores are abundant in urban and rural areas, yet usually carry little healthy food. The cost of purchasing new refrigerators and sinks in which to prepare and store perishable items is often prohibitive for many small store owners. Fear of unsold or spoiled stock may also contribute to their reluctance to purchase perishable food inventory. Finding ways around these barriers could benefit both consumers and storeowners. Finally, the effect of the recession on consumer food choice and store survival may require more clarification, because the state of the economy is uncertain.

Development of a method to assess total cost, to include price, food access, preparation time, and convenience, would assist in understanding the situation in a particular community and ways to improve it.

Social Sciences

The social, cultural, and psychological factors that influence human behavior are clearly relevant to explain how consumers interact with the food environment. The most effective interventions will be those that are sensitive to the needs of diverse populations.

On the supply side, in addition to the economic issues, there may also be a psychological component to why supermarket executives are reluctant to site stores in food deserts and why a store does not want to be the first of its kind in a neighborhood. This is in contrast to their UK counterparts that seem to be more willing partners in regenerating urban stores. If data can back up this perception, perhaps more targeted policies can ensue.

Psychosocial factors that affect small-store owners and shoppers are also important to explore, such as feelings of self-esteem, stress, and locus of control. As examples, these factors may affect how store owners and employees interact with customers, as well as how willing customers are to purchase and prepare healthy foods that might be new to them. The roles that food venues play in the community and for individuals go beyond places for commercial transactions.

Urban Planning

The public health implications of zoning and transportation are additional areas in which urban planners can contribute their expertise. The lack of transportation to existing stores is an issue for some because people do not have the means to travel outside food deserts, yet the population may be too small and dispersed to support new markets. This is an area of study where urban planners could help develop useful approaches to improving transportation infrastructure so that those lacking private transportation could gain access.

The current planning paradigm favors mixed-use "smart growth," an urban planning concept that clusters growth in the center of a city to create more walkable, lively neighborhoods and urban areas. Still to be understood is the role the food environment plays in where people choose to live and how smart growth affects health.

Policy

Policy makers could use the available findings to develop policies at federal, state, and local levels that are intended to improve dietary behavior while recognizing that many unknowns may affect final outcomes. Some of the policies identified in the workshop that will benefit from filling research gaps include the following:

- How federal and other government benefit programs can encourage healthier eating;
- The effect of taxing unhealthy food (especially sweetened beverages) and/or subsidizing healthy food; and

- The best mix of financial and other incentives to site supermarkets in food deserts and to encourage existing stores to stock healthy items.

In concert with additional research, it is important to connect conceptual data with the context of people's everyday lives and to fully explore the consequences, often unintended, of decisions around such a pervasive, personal issue as food choice.

NEXT STEPS AND CLOSING THOUGHTS

Improvements in the methodology of food desert research will be helpful for developing evidence-based, locally appropriate interventions. The interplay between supply and demand is complex. Many workshop participants expressed that a supply of healthy food needs to be available and affordable for consumers to purchase and prepare on a regular basis. However, focusing only on supply, especially when healthy items cost relatively more than less healthy options, may not have a significant impact on the health of individuals or broader communities; consumer demand—in the forms of preferences and knowledge—also affects consumption decisions and subsequently health outcomes. In addition, a caveat ran throughout the workshop that retail is but one part of a larger food environment in which both healthy and less healthy choices abound. Consumers get food messages from sources that range from the media, to family and friends, schools and other educational outlets, and underlying cultural norms. Businesses operate on thin profit margins and they constantly balance customer demand for both healthy and less healthy (but often good-tasting) choices.

To close the workshop, Barry Popkin, planning committee chair, thanked staff, speakers, and participants. Understanding food deserts is the beginning of a long set of issues to understand how to improve the diets of Americans.

References

Auchincloss, A.H., A.V. Diez Roux, M. Shen, A.G. Bertoni, M.R. Carnethon, and M.S. Mujahid. Unpublished. Do people living in neighborhoods with good resources for being physically active and eating healthy foods have lower risk of type 2 diabetes (the Multi-Ethnic Study of Atherosclerosis)? Under review.

Ayala, G. 2009. Unpublished. Working with tiendas to promote healthy eating. Presented at the Institute of Medicine-National Research Council Workshop on the Public Health Effects of Food Deserts, Washington, DC, January 26-27.

Beaulac, J., E. Kristjansson, and S. Cummins. In press. Food deserts. A systematic review (1966-2007). *Preventing Chronic Disease.*

Berkey, C.S., H.R.H. Rockett, W.C. Willett, and G.A. Colditz. 2005. Milk, dairy fat, dietary calcium, and weight gain: A longitudinal study of adolescents. *Archives of Pediatrics & Adolescent Medicine* 159:543-550.

Beydoun, M.A., T.L. Gary, B.H. Caballero, R.S. Lawrence, L.J. Cheskin, and Y. Wang. 2008. Ethnic differences in dairy and related nutrient consumption among U.S. adults and their association with obesity, central obesity, and the metabolic syndrome. *American Journal of Clinical Nutrition* 87:1914-1925.

Blanck, H. 2009. Unpublished. Farmer's Markets. Discussion at the Institute of Medicine-National Research Council Workshop on the Public Health Effects of Food Deserts, Washington, DC, January 26-27.

Cummins, S. 2009. Unpublished. Understanding the environmental determinants of diet: A geographical perspective. Presented at the Institute of Medicine-National Research Council Workshop on the Public Health Effects of Food Deserts, Washington, DC, January 26-27.

Cummins, S., M. Pettigrew, C. Higgins, A. Findlay, and L. Sparks. 2005. Large scale food retailing as an intervention for diet and health: Quasi-experimental evaluation of a natural experiment. *Journal of Epidemiology and Community Health* 59:1035-1040.

Duffey, K.J., and B.M. Popkin. 2007. Shifts in patterns and consumption of beverages between 1965 and 2002. *Obesity* 15:2739-2747.

Duffey, K.J., P. Gordon-Larsen, G.X. Ayala, and B.M. Popkin. 2008. Birthplace is associated with more adverse dietary profiles for U.S. versus foreign born Latino adults. *Journal of Nutrition* 138:2428-2435.

Franco, M., A.V. Diez Roux, T.A. Glass, B. Caballero, and F.L. Brancati. 2008. Neighborhood characteristics and availability of healthy foods in Baltimore. *American Journal of Preventive Medicine* 35:561.

Franco, M., A.V. Diez Roux, J.A. Nettleton, M. Lazo, F. Brancati, B. Caballero, T. Glass, and L.V. Moore. 2009. Availability of healthy foods and dietary patterns: The Multi-Ethnic Study of Atherosclerosis. *America Journal of Clinical Nutrition* 89:1-7.

French, S.A., R.W. Jeffrey, M. Story, K.K. Breitlow, J.S. Baxter, P. Hannan, and M.P. Snyder. 2001. Pricing and promotion effects of low-fat vending snack purchases: The CHIPS study. *American Journal of Public Health* 91:112-117.

Gallagher, M. 2009. Unpublished. Measuring food deserts. Presented at the Institute of Medicine-National Research Council Workshop on the Public Health Effects of Food Deserts, Washington, DC, January 26-27.

Glanz, K., J.F. Sallis, B.E. Saelens, and L.D. Frank. 2005. Healthy nutrition environments: Concepts and measures. *American Journal of Health Promotion* 19:330-333.

Guagliardo, M.F. 2004. Spatial accessibility of primary care: Concepts, methods and challenges. *International Journal of Health Geographics* 3:3.

He, K., F.B. Hu, G.A. Colditz, J.E. Manson, W.C. Willett, and S. Liu. 2004. Changes in intake of fruits and vegetables in relation to risk of obesity and weight gain among middle-aged women. *International Journal of Obesity* 28:1569-1574.

Hu, F.B., and W.C. Willett. 2002. Optimal diets for prevention of coronary heart disease. *Journal of the American Medical Association* 288:2569-2578.

Hu, F.B., M.J. Stampfer, J.E. Manson, E. Rimm, G.A. Colditz, B.A. Rosner, C.H. Hennekens, and W.C. Willett. 1997. Dietary fat intake and the risk of coronary heart disease in women. *New England Journal of Medicine* 337:1491-1499.

Khan, A.A., and S.M. Bhardwaj. 1994. Access to health care: A conceptual framework and its relevance to health care planning. *Evaluation & the Health Professions* 17:60-76.

Kling, J.R., J.B. Liebman, and L.F. Katz. 2007. Experimental analysis of neighborhood effects. *Econometrica* 75:83-119.

Leibtag, E. 2009. Unpublished. Dynamics of the food shopping environment. Presented at the Institute of Medicine-National Research Council Workshop on the Public Health Effects of Food Deserts, Washington, DC, January 26-27.

Liu, S., W.C. Willett, M.J. Stampfer, F.B. Hu, M. Franz, L. Sampson, C.H. Hennekens, and J.E. Manson. 2000. A prospective study of dietary glycemic load, carbohydrate intake, and risk of coronary heart disease in U.S. women. *American Journal of Clinical Nutrition* 71:1455-1461.

Liu, S., W.C. Willett, J.E. Manson, F.B. Hu, B. Rosner, and G.A. Colditz. 2003. Relation between changes in intakes of dietary fiber and grain products and changes in weight and development of obesity among middle-aged women. *American Journal of Clinical Nutrition* 78:920-927.

Macintyre, S. 2007. Deprivation amplification revisited; or, is it always true that poorer places have poorer access to resources for healthy diets and physical activity? *International Journal of Behavioral Nutrition and Physical Activity* 4:32.

Mattes, R. 2009. Unpublished. Effects of selected dietary factors on obesity. Presented at the Institute of Medicine-National Research Council Workshop on the Public Health Effects of Food Deserts, Washington, DC, January 26-27.

Moore, L.V., and A.V. Diez Roux. 2006. Associations of neighborhood characteristics with the location and type of food stores. *American Journal of Public Health* 96:325-331.

Moore, L.V., A.V. Diez Roux, J.A. Nettleton, and D.R. Jacobs, Jr. 2008. Associations of the local food environment with diet quality—A comparison of assessments based on surveys and geographic information systems: The Multi-Ethnic Study of Atherosclerosis. *American Journal of Epidemiology* 167:917-924.

Nonas, C. 2009. Unpublished. New York City: Healthy food access. Presented at the Institute of Medicine-National Research Council Workshop on the Public Health Effects of Food Deserts, Washington, DC, January 26-27.

Popkin, B. 2009. Unpublished. Workshop on the Public Health Effects of Food Deserts. Presented at the Institute of Medicine-National Research Council Workshop on the Public Health Effects of Food Deserts, Washington, DC, January 26-27.

Powell, L.M., and Y. Bao. In press. Food prices, access to food outlets and child weight. *Economics & Human Biology.*

Powell, L.M., S. Slater, D. Mirtcheva, Y. Bao, and F.J. Chaloupka. 2007. Food store availability and neighborhood characteristics in the United States. *Preventive Medicine* 44:189-195.

Schulze, M.B., J.E. Manson, D.S. Ludwig, G.A. Colditz, M.J. Stampfer, W.C. Willett, and F.B. Hu. 2004. Sugar-sweetened beverages, weight gain, and incidence of Type 2 diabetes in young and middle-aged women. *Journal of the American Medical Association* 292:927-934.

Seymour, J.D., A.L. Yaroch, M. Serdula, H.M. Blanck, and L.K. Khan. 2004. Impact of nutrition and environmental interventions on point-of-purchase behavior in adults: A review. *Preventive Medicine* 39:S108-S136.

SFC (Sustainable Food Center). 1995. *Access denied: An analysis of problems facing East Austin residents in their attempts to obtain affordable, nutritious food.* Austin, TX.

Sharkey, J. 2009. Unpublished. Rural food deserts: Perspective from rural Texas. Presented at the Institute of Medicine-National Research Council Workshop on the Public Health Effects of Food Deserts, Washington, DC, January 26-27.

Song, Y., and G.J. Knaap. 2003. New urbanism and housing values: A disaggregated assessment. *Journal of Urban Economics* 54:218-238.

Song, Y., and G.J. Knaap. 2004. Measuring the effects of mixed land uses on housing values. *Regional Science and Urban Economics* 34:663-680.

Song, Y., and J. Sohn. 2007. Valuing spatial accessibility to retailing: A case study of the single family housing market in Hillsboro, Oregon. *Journal of Retailing and Consumer Services* 14:279-288.

Sturm, R., and A. Datar. 2005. Body mass index in elementary school children, metropolitan area food prices and food outlet density. *Public Health* 119:1059-1068.

Sturm, R., and A. Datar. 2008. Food prices and weight gain during elementary school: 5-year update. *Public Health* 122:1140-1143.

Tropp, D. 2009. Unpublished. Farmer's Markets. Discussion at the Institute of Medicine-National Research Council Workshop on the Public Health Effects of Food Deserts, Washington, DC, January 26-27.

USDA (U.S. Department of Agriculture) ERS (Economic Research Service). 2000. Beverages. Available online at http://www.ers.usda.gov/Data/FoodConsumption/FoodAvail Spreadsheets.htm [accessed January 2003].

USDA NASS (National Agricultural Statistics Survey). 2009. 2007 Census of Agriculture. Census of Agriculture. Volume I, Part 51. United States. Summary and State Data.

Wrigley, N., D. Warm, and B. Margetts. 2003. Deprivation, diet and food retail access: Findings from the Leeds "Food Deserts" study. *Environment and Planning A* 35:151-188.

Appendix A

Planning Committee Biographies

Barry M. Popkin, Ph.D. (*Chair*), is the Carla Steel Chamblee Distinguished Professor of Global Nutrition at the University of North Carolina, Chapel Hill, where he directs the Interdisciplinary Center for Obesity. Dr. Popkin has an active U.S. research program in understanding dietary behavior with a focus on eating patterns, trends, and sociodemographic determinants; the nutrition transition and the rapid changes in obesity; dynamic changes in diet, physical activity, and inactivity; body composition changes (and the factors responsible for these changes); consequences of these changes; and program and policy options for managing change. He is active in research in the United States, as well as in studies of countries around the world funded by the National Institutes of health (NIH), including detailed longitudinal studies that he directs in China and Russia. His U.S. work includes a series of NIH grants to study how socioeconomic change linked to shifts in the built environment affects diet, activity, and obesity in the Add Health and a second 20-year long longitudinal study—CARDIA.

Ana V. Diez Roux, M.D., M.P.H., Ph.D., is professor of epidemiology, director of the Center for Integrative Approaches to Health Disparities, and associate director of the Center for Social Epidemiology and Population Health at the University of Michigan. Dr. Diez Roux is an epidemiologist whose work has focused on the examination of the social determinants of health. Her empirical work has focused on the social determinants of cardiovascular disease with special emphasis on the examination of how residential environments shape the distribution of cardiovascular risk. She has also published on multilevel analysis and on the methodological challenges faced by epidemiology as it integrates population-level and individual-level determinants in understanding the causes of disease. Recent work also focuses on the role of air pollution exposures and psychosocial stress. Dr. Diez-Roux has been an international leader in the application of multilevel analysis in epidemiology and in the investigation of neighborhood health effects.

Joel Gittelsohn, Ph.D., is associate professor of international health at Johns Hopkins University. He is a medical anthropologist who specializes in the use of qualitative and quantitative information to design, implement, and evaluate health and nutrition intervention programs. Dr. Gittelsohn integrates both qualitative and quantitative approaches to better understand culture-based beliefs and behaviors regarding dietary patterns, and how these factors influence the success or failure of dietary and lifestyle modification strategies. He applies these methods and interventions for the prevention of obesity and diabetes among different indigenous and ethnic groups, to nutrient deficiencies of Nepalese children and women, and to improve infant feeding in diverse settings. He is currently working on chronic disease interventions among the White Mountain and San Carlos Apache (obesity prevention), the Ojibwa-Cree (diabetes prevention), African-American churchgoing women (cardiovascular disease prevention), and children and adults in the Republic of the Marshall Islands (prevention of obesity and undernutrition).

Barbara A. Laraia, M.P.H., Ph.D., R.D., is assistant professor in the Department of Medicine at the University of California, San Francisco, and co-director of COAST. Dr. Laraia is a public health nutrition investigator with a special interest in the relationships between food policy, the food environment, and health. She has expertise in qualitative methods, program evaluation, community-based research, and nutritional epidemiology. Her research focuses on household food security status and neighborhood effects on diet, weight, perinatal outcomes, and other maternal and child health issues, especially among vulnerable populations. Her current projects include measurement issues of the food and physical activity environments; influences of the food environment on diet and weight among postpartum women; and understanding the role that tiendas (Latino grocery stores) play in diet quality among Latinos.

Robin A. McKinnon, M.P.A., Ph.D., is health policy specialist at the National Cancer Institute. Dr. McKinnon works on activities intended to advance policy-relevant research on diet, physical activity, and weight.

Her research interests focus on public policies intended to reduce obesity incidence and prevalence and include: The effects of food and physical activity environments on individual diet and physical activity behavior, measurement of the food and physical activity environments, and the economic and societal effects of increased obesity rates. Dr. McKinnon earned her Ph.D. in public policy and administration at the George Washington University in Washington, DC. She also received a master of public administration from Harvard University, and a bachelor of arts degree from the Australian National University.

Joseph R. Sharkey, M.P.H., Ph.D., R.D., is associate professor of sociology in the School of Rural Public Health (SRPH) at Texas A&M University System Health Science Center. He is also director of the Texas Healthy Aging Research Network (TxHAN) and director of the Program for Research in Nutrition and Health Disparities, SRPH. One of his current research projects, "Behavioral and Environmental Influence on Obesity: Rural Context & Race/Ethnicity," aims to examine the interplay of behavioral (individual and family) and environmental (home, social, and neighborhood-community) factors, food choice, and healthful eating among African-American, Hispanic, and non-Hispanic white families of rural Central Texas. The study will use a mixed-methods approach that includes qualitative (key informant interviews, focus groups, and participant observations), quantitative (in-home surveys and household food audits), and geographic information system (GIS) technology research methods.

Appendix B

Workshop Agenda

Workshop on the Public Health Effects of Food Deserts
January 26-27, 2009

Keck Center of The National Academies
500 Fifth Street, N.W., Washington, DC
Keck 100

Monday, January 26

8:00 a.m.   Registration and check-in

8:30-8:40   Welcome and introductory remarks
               Barry Popkin, Planning committee chair

8:40-9:00   Congressionally mandated study of food deserts: Work
               of the U.S. Department of Agriculture (USDA) Economic
               Research Service
               *Laurian Unnevehr and Shelly Ver Ploeg, USDA Economic
               Research Service*

9:00-9:10   Overview of workshop
               Barry Popkin, Chair

SESSION 1: **Measuring "food deserts": Demography and
                the dynamics of food accessibility, availability,
                affordability, and quality**

9:10-9:30   National overview of demographics and socioeconomic
               status
               Lisa Powell, University of Illinois at Chicago

9:30-9:50   Urban food deserts: Perspective from Chicago and Detroit
               *Mari Gallagher, Mari Gallagher Research and Consulting
               Group*

9:50-10:10   Rural food deserts: Perspective from rural Texas
               Joseph Sharkey, Texas A&M University

10:10-10:30   The current and future dynamics of the food shopping
               environment
               Ephraim Leibtag, USDA Economic Research Service

10:30-10:45   Break

10:45-11:45   Moderated Panel Discussion
               *Moderator: Heidi Blanck, Centers for Disease Control and
               Prevention (CDC) National Center for Chronic Disease
               Prevention & Health Promotion*

11:45-1:00   Lunch on your own

SESSION 2: **Challenges in identifying causal effects of food
               environment on health**

1:00-1:20   A view from an epidemiological approach
               Ana Diez Roux, University of Michigan

1:20-1:40   A view from a geospatial approach
               Steven Cummins, University of London

1:40-2:00   A view from an economic approach
               Yan Song, University of North Carolina at Chapel Hill

2:00-2:45   Moderated Panel Discussion
               *Moderator: Jill Reedy, National Cancer Institute, National
               Institutes of Health (NIH)*

2:45-3:00   Public Comment Period

3:00-3:15   Break

SESSION 3:   **The potential health consequences of changes to diet**

3:15-3:35   Effects of select dietary factors on obesity
              Richard Mattes, Purdue University

3:35-3:55   Effects of select dietary factors on cardiovascular diseases
              and cancer
              Frank Hu, Harvard School of Public Health

3:55-4:45   Moderated Panel Discussion
              Moderator: Wendy Johnson-Askew, National Institute of
              Diabetes and Digestive and Kidney Diseases, NIH

4:45-5:00   Wrap-up for the day
              Barry Popkin, Chair

5:00   Adjourn

5:00-6:00   Conversation and light refreshments

Tuesday, January 27

8:00 a.m.   Registration and check-in

8:30-8:40   Welcome and overview of day 2 of the workshop
              Barry Popkin, Planning committee chair

SESSION 4:   **Changing food deserts: Lessons from current**
                 intervention research

8:40-9:00   Overview of efforts to change the food environment
              Joel Gittelsohn, Johns Hopkins University

9:00-9:20   Effect of introducing new supermarkets
              Neil Wrigley, University of Southampton

9:20-9:40   Intervening in small Hispanic grocery stores (tiendas)
              Guadalupe "Suchi" Ayala, San Diego State University

9:40-9:50   Break to set up videoconference

9:50-10:10   Developing and supporting farmers markets
                Andrew Smiley, Sustainable Food Center (via videoconference)

10:10-10:30   Break

10:30-11:30   Moderated Panel Discussion
                *Moderator: Terry Huang, National Institute of Child Health
                and Human Development, NIH*

11:30-1:00   Lunch on your own

SESSION 5: **Policy and program options to increase food
                accessibility in a dynamic food environment**

1:00-1:15   Top-down approach—New York as a case study
                *Cathy Nonas, New York City Department of Health & Mental
                Hygiene*

1:15-1:30   Bottom-up approach
                John Weidman, The Food Trust

1:30-1:45   Community-level food environment
                Andy Fisher, Food Security Coalition

1:45-2:00   Evaluation of the SNAP (Supplemental Nutrition
                Assistance Program) and WIC (Women, Infants, and
                Children) pilot program changes
                August Schumacher, Jr., Kellogg Foundation

2:00-2:15   How do grocers site store locations?
                Bill Drake, Cornell University

2:15-2:30   Break

2:30-3:15   Moderated Panel Discussion
                Moderator: Robin McKinnon, National Cancer Institute, NIH

3:15-3:45   Break

SESSION 6:   Research gaps and needs

(To provide input about gaps and future research needs, please submit notecards to staff by 2:30 p.m. prior to the panel discussion in session 5.)

3:45-4:15   Summary of research gaps and needs discussed
                at workshop and standards needed for evaluating
                interventions
                Robin McKinnon, National Cancer Institute, NIH

4:15-4:30   Closing remarks
                Barry Popkin, Chair

4:30   Adjourn

Appendix C

Speaker and Moderator Biographies

Guadalupe X. "Suchi" Ayala is an associate professor in the Division of Health Promotion in the Graduate School of Public Health, San Diego State University. She is co-principal investigator (co-PI) of the San Diego Prevention Research Center and a co-investigator on the Hispanic Community Health Study (Proyecto SOL). Dr. Ayala's primary areas of research include: (1) examining sociocultural and environmental determinants of Latino health, specifically diet, physical activity, and risk of overweight and obesity; and (2) developing family- and community-based interventions to promote Latino health, including working with tiendas to promote healthy eating. She has received more than 10 grants as a PI, including funding from the National Cancer Institute, the Centers for Disease Control and Prevention (CDC), the American Cancer Society, and the United States Department of Agriculture (USDA), which have resulted in 41 manuscripts and 9 book chapters.

Heidi Blanck is the team lead for Nutrition Research and Surveillance at the CDC in the Division of Nutrition, Physical Activity, and Obesity. Dr. Blanck is an epidemiologist and oversees CDC's monitoring of nutrition behavior and environmental and policy supports for fruits and vegetables and breastfeeding target areas. Her research interests include the effects of the environment on individual dietary behavior, measurement of the community and consumer food environment, and policies intended to improve access to healthy foods. She coordinates the State Food Environment Workgroup, a forum for states and researchers to share food environment tools. She also serves on the planning committee for the upcoming Food Systems and Public Health Meeting and on the National Collaborative on Childhood Obesity Research (NCCOR) Policy Surveillance Workgroup. Her current projects include a population-based assessment of American's perceptions of affordability, access, and availability of fruits and vegetables and assessment of state policies intended to improve the access and availability of fruits and vegetables.

Steven Cummins is a geographer with training in epidemiology and public health. He is currently senior lecturer and National Institute for Health Research (NIHR) fellow in the Department of Geography, Queen Mary, University of London, where he leads the Healthy Environments Research Programme. Dr. Cummins' primary research interests are in the contextual and socioenvironmental determinants of health and the design and evaluation of community social and policy interventions to improve population health. He is currently a member of the UK Food Standards Agency Social Science Research Committee and the NIHR Public Health Research Programme Funding Board. In 2007, he was awarded a Philip Leverhulme Prize for his work on the socioenvironmental determinants of health.

Bill Drake is a senior extension associate and director of executive education with the Food Industry Management Program (FIMP) at Cornell University. Mr. Drake developed and directs the National Association of Convenience Stores Leadership Executive Program and the National Grocers Association Executive Leadership Program. In addition, he teaches in the Food Executive Program, United Fresh Executive Leadership Program, and FIMP's various international food executive programs. Prior to Cornell, Mr. Drake spent 20 years as an executive with SuperValu Inc., a large U.S. food retailer.

Andy Fisher is co-founder and executive director of the Community Food Security Coalition (CFSC), a national association of 260 organizations working to create a just and sustainable food system. CFSC has spearheaded the development of a national food and farming movement centered on connecting farmers and consumers and improving access to healthy foods in low-income communities. Mr. Fisher is a leading expert in the field of food security and has coauthored numerous articles and studies on the topic. He has served on the board of the National Campaign for Sustainable Agriculture and the California Sustainable Agriculture Working Group. He holds graduate degrees from the University of California at Los Angeles (UCLA) in environmental policy and Latin American studies.

Mari Gallagher is president of the Mari Gallagher Research & Consulting Group and the newly formed National Center for Public Research. Ms. Gallagher authored *Examining the Impact of Food Deserts on Public Health in Chicago*, a breakthrough study that popularized the term "food desert" nationally and encouraged Congressman Bobby Rush to enter food desert language into the Farm Bill. She was the first to develop a block-by-block metric for food deserts and food balance linked with health measures and has since done similar work in Detroit; rural Michigan; Louisville, Kentucky; Harlem; Richmond, Virginia; and other areas.

Frank Hu is professor of nutrition and epidemiology at the Harvard School of Public Health. He also serves as director of the Boston Obesity and Nutrition Research Center Epidemiology and Genetics Core. His research is focused primarily on epidemiology and prevention of Type 2 diabetes and metabolic diseases through diet and lifestyle. He is also interested in gene-environment interactions in relation to obesity, Type 2 diabetes, and cardiovascular complications.

Terry Huang is director of the Obesity Research Strategic Core at the Eunice Kennedy Shriver National Institute of Child Health and Human Development (NICHHD), National Institutes of Health (NIH). Dr. Huang plays a major role in developing new research directions and funding priorities in the area of pediatric obesity at the NICHHD and across the NIH. He is currently leading an agenda on global multilevel research in pediatric obesity and has special interest in society-biology interactions in obesity and chronic disease, multilevel prevention strategies, international health, pediatric metabolic syndrome, fetal and childhood antecedents of obesity and metabolic abnormalities, and the translation of science to policy in the prevention of obesity and chronic disease. Dr. Huang is a fellow of the Obesity Society (TOS) and councilor on the Pediatric Obesity Section of TOS. In addition, he serves on the Senior Leadership Group of the NIH Obesity Research Task Force and represents the NICHHD nationally and internationally on panels related to pediatric obesity. Dr. Huang received his Ph.D. in preventive medicine and M.P.H. in epidemiology and biostatistics from the University of Southern California. Prior to joining the NIH, he served on the faculty of the University of Kansas Medical Center and Tufts University's Friedman School of Nutrition Science and Policy.

Wendy Johnson-Askew is public health nutrition and health policy adviser for the Division of Nutrition Research Coordination within the National Institutes of Health. Prior to coming to NIH, Dr. Johnson-Askew held a number of clinical nutrition management positions and nutrition faculty positions. Dr. Johnson-Askew received her Ph.D. and M.P.H. degrees from the School of Public Health at the University of North Carolina at Chapel Hill. Her areas of research interest include community nutrition intervention strategies, community efforts to reduce or eliminate health disparities, effective nutrition communication strategies, and community-based anti-hunger efforts. Dr. Johnson-Askew has been actively involved in follow-up actions to the Surgeon General's Call to Action to Prevent and Decrease Overweight and Obesity, and she speaks to a wide variety of audiences on the topic.

Ephraim Leibtag is a senior economist with USDA's Economic Research Service. He researches retail food prices and the dynamics of retail food markets. His research interests include tracking, forecasting, and analyzing trends in retail food markets, and his work is used in presentations to government officials, policy analysts, the research community, and other public audiences. Dr. Leibtag has conducted television, radio, and newspaper interviews on retail food price trends. He has M.A. and Ph.D. degrees in economics from the University of Maryland.

Richard Mattes is professor of foods and nutrition at Purdue University, adjunct associate professor of medicine at the Indiana University School of Medicine, and affiliated scientist at the Monell Chemical Senses Center. His research focuses on the areas of hunger and satiety, regulation of food intake in humans, food preferences, human cephalic phase responses, and taste and smell. At Purdue University, Dr. Mattes is the director of the Ingestive Behavior Research Center; director of the Analytical Core Laboratory for the Botanical Center for Age-Related Diseases, and chair of the Human Subjects Review Committee. Dr. Mattes earned an undergraduate degree in biology and a master's degree in public health from the University of Michigan as well as a doctorate degree in human nutrition from Cornell University. He conducted postdoctoral studies at the Memorial Sloan-Kettering Cancer Center and the Monell Chemical Senses Center.

Cathy Nonas is director of Physical Activity and Nutrition Programs for the New York City Department of Health & Mental Hygiene. A clinical dietitian by training, she has a long history in working with and writing about patients with obesity and Type 2 diabetes, both at the federally funded Obesity Research Center and as assistant clinical professor at Mt. Sinai School of Medicine. Concerned that good treatment techniques are not sustainable within an environment that promotes obesity, for the last two years she has been working on policy changes to increase access to healthy foods in underserved neighborhoods and create opportunities for physical activity for young children. Changes in daycare regulations, permitting of 1,000 fresh fruit and vegetable vendors for city streets, and calorie posting in chain restaurants are some of the policies she has been working on.

Lisa Powell is senior research scientist in the Institute for Health Research and Policy and research associate professor in the Department of Economics at the University of Illinois at Chicago. Dr. Powell has extensive experience as an applied microeconomist in the empirical analysis of the effects of public policy on a series of behavioral outcomes. As director of the ImpacTeen Youth Obesity Research Team funded by the Robert Wood Johnson Foundation (RWJF) and as principal investigator on a Nutritional Research Initiative (NRI) USDA-funded project, much of her current research is on assessing the importance of economic and environmental factors (such as food prices and access to food stores, eating places, and parks, gyms, and other facilities for physical activity) on food consumption and physical activity behaviors and as determinants of body mass index (BMI) and the prevalence of obesity. Dr. Powell's research also examines school-level food and fitness policies and the association of school meal participation and children's weight status. In other health-related work, Dr. Powell has examined the importance of peer and parental influences on teen smoking, while other studies have highlighted the role of prices and public policies with regard to alcohol use among college students and educational and violence-related outcomes.

Jill Reedy is a program director at the National Cancer Institute in the Risk Factor Monitoring and Methods Branch in the Applied Research Program. She is a program lead for the Diet and Physical Activity Program of NIH's Genes, Environment, and Health Initiative—this program aims to develop innovative technologies to measure diet and physical activity in large-scale population studies. Dr. Reedy is a nutritionist whose research focuses on dietary patterning, dietary assessment, dietary monitoring, and the food environment. She is currently working on a comparison of different methodological approaches in dietary pattern analysis (including factor analysis, cluster analysis, and index analysis) and an ongoing compilation of measures of the food environment (available at https:// riskfactor.cancer.gov/mfe).

August Schumacher, Jr., is adviser to SJH and Company and consultant with the Kellogg Foundation. He is the former under secretary for Farm and Foreign Agricultural Services at USDA. He was responsible for the domestic commodities, insurance, and farm credit operations of USDA. In addition, he was in charge of USDA's international trade and development programs. Prior to his appointment in August 1997, he was the administrator of the Foreign Agricultural Service for three years. Before coming to USDA, Mr. Schumacher served as commissioner of the Massachusetts Department of Food and Agriculture and as a senior agricultural project officer at the World Bank. From a farm family in Lexington, Massachusetts, Mr. Schumacher attended Harvard College and the London School of Economics, and was a research associate in agribusiness at the Harvard Business School.

Andrew W. Smiley has more than 15 years' experience working in sustainable agriculture and food systems, including on-farm production, agricultural marketing, micro-enterprise development, food journalism, farmer training and technical assistance, and even food service management. Mr. Smiley received his B.A. in political science from Louisiana State University in Baton Rouge. He is the former executive director of Baton Rouge Economic and Agricultural Development Alliance, Inc. (BREADA). Andrew is an active supporter and volunteer of the Southern Sustainable Agriculture Working Group (Southern SAWG) and Texas Organic Farmers and Gardeners Association (TOFGA), and has applied his passion for organic gardening, sustainable food systems, small-scale farming, and healthy cooking to his work with Sustainable Food Center since 2005. Andrew currently works with Sustainable Food Center in Austin, Texas, as farm projects director, which includes management of several farm marketing and food systems education initiatives, including Sprouting Healthy Kids—SFC's farm-to-school pilot project.

Yan Song is assistant professor in the Department of City and Regional Planning at the University of North Carolina. Dr. Song's research areas include urban spatial structure, location choice of households and residents, smart growth and urban growth management, comparative evaluations of urban development, and urban system modeling. Dr. Song has published extensively in journals such as the *Journal of Urban Economics, Regional Science and Urban Economics, Journal of American Planning Association, Urban Studies,* and *Journal of Regional Science.* Her articles have regularly been among the top-downloaded articles from these journals.

John Weidman works closely with the executive director, the founder, and the senior staff of the Food Trust to oversee all programs and provide strong leadership for the organization. He develops and advances public policies at the local, state, and federal levels; and educates local, state, and federal policy makers about the factors impacting the nutrition of lower-income people. John oversees a comprehensive communications strategy, and he provided executive leadership in the successful start-up of the Headhouse Farmers' Market, Philadelphia's largest open-air farmers market. John has 15 years of experience in public policy advocacy and nonprofit communications. He holds a master's degree in political science from the University of Pennsylvania.

Neil Wrigley is professor of geography, University of Southampton, UK, and editor of the *Journal of Economic Geography* (Oxford University Press). He is an economic geographer whose research over the past 15 years has focused on issues of retailing and consumption but who is also widely known for his earlier contributions to quantitative social science. During 1999-2003, together with colleagues in public health, he conducted and published pioneering research on issues of food poverty, diet-related health inequalities, and food retail access in underserved low-income neighborhoods of British cities. In particular, his Economic and Social Research Council (ESRC) Leeds food deserts study provided one of the first attempts to assess the consequences of the amelioration of access problems in an unsupportive local food environment following the opening of one of the UK's initial urban regeneration-focused supermarkets. Dr. Wrigley is academician of the Academy of Social Sciences; served for eight years as a member of the Research Resources & Methods Committee of the UK Economic & Social Research Council; has held Leverhulme, ESRC, and Erskine fellowships; and was senior research fellow, St. Peter's College, Oxford. Among several prizes he has received, he was most recently awarded the Royal Geographical Society's Murchison Award 2008 for his publications on the geographies of retailing and consumption.

Appendix D

Workshop Participants

Jennifer Abel, Virginia Cooperative Extension
Mariela Alarcon-Yohe, Directors of Health Promotion and Education
Guadalupe Ayala, San Diego State University
Lindsey Baker, Feeding America
Jodi Balis, Capital Area Food Bank
Neil Bania, University of Oregon
Jim Barham, United States Department of Agriculture
Heidi Blanck, Centers for Disease Control and Prevention
Daniel Block, Chicago State University
Covington Brown, Summit Health Institute of Research and Education
Erin Caricofe, Northeast Midwest Institute
Judith Chambers, Emerging Market Solutions
Susan E. Chen, Purdue University
Kay Cherry, Eastern Virginia Medical School
Cindy Chiou, Urban Design Lab at the Earth Institute at Columbia
    University
Dan Christenson, U.S. Senate Committee on Agriculture, Nutrition &
    Forestry
Andrea Collier, W.K. Kellogg Foundation Food and Society Policy
    Fellow
Steven Cummins, University of London
Valerie Darcey, Drexel University
Judith Dausch, American Heart Association
Adam Diamond, United States Department of Agriculture

Lorelei DiSogra, United Fresh Produce Association
Karen Donato, National Heart, Lung, and Blood Institute, National
    Institutes of Health
William Drake, Cornell University
Megan Elsener, Food Research and Action Center
Christa Essig, Centers for Disease Control and Prevention
Jessie Fan, University of Utah
Tracey Farrigan, United States Department of Agriculture, Economic
    Research Service
Andy Fisher, Community Food Security Coalition
Rachel Fisher, National Institutes of Health
Paula Ford, Kansas State University
Mari Gallagher, Mari Gallagher Research & Consulting Group
Karen Glanz, Emory University
Sonya Grier, American University
Barbara Harrison, Affliation Unknown
Arnell Hinkle, California Adolescent Nutrition and Fitness
Frank Hu, Harvard School of Public Health
Terry Huang, National Institutes of Health
Wendy Johnson-Askew, National Institutes of Health
Eugene Kim, Affliation Unknown
Kelly Kinnison, United States Department of Agriculture, Food and
    Nutrition Service
Rebecca Klein, Johns Hopkins Center for a Livable Future
Vivica Kraak, Save the Children
Michael LeBlanc, United States Department of Agriculture, Economic
    Research Service
Laura Leete, University of Oregon
Ephraim Leibtag, United States Department of Agriculture, Economic
    Research Service
Angela Liese, University of South Carolina
Richard Mattes, Purdue University
Meredith McGehee, California WIC Association
Ruth Morgan, Altarum Institute
Kelly Morrison, World Hunger Year
Annie Moss, Montefiore School Health Program
Suzanne Murphy, University of Hawaii
Kathryn Neckerman, Columbia University
Ronnie Neff, Johns Hopkins Bloomberg School of Public Health
Jonathan Nomachi, Community Health Councils
Cathy Nonas, New York City Department of Health & Mental Hygiene
Julie Obbagy, N. Chapman Associates
Lisa Marie Powell, University of Illinois at Chicago

Rose Pribilovics, Summit Health Institute of Research and Education
Marnie Purciel, Columbia University
Jill Reedy, National Cancer Institute
August Schumacher, Kellogg Foundation
Naomi Senkeeto, American Diabetes Association
Andrew Smiley, Sustainable Food Center
Robert Andrew Smith, The Leaflight, Inc.
Yan Song, University of North Carolina at Chapel Hill
Andrea Sparks, United States Department of Housing and Urban
    Development
Kathryn Strong, Physicians Committee for Responsible Medicine
Linda Thompson, Howard University
Sarah Treuhaft, PolicyLink
Debra Tropp, United States Department of Agriculture, Agricultural
    Marketing Service
Elizabeth Tuckermanty, United States Department of Agriculture,
    Cooperative State Research, Education, and Extension Service
Laurian Unnevehr, United States Department of Agriculture, Economic
    Research Service
Shelly Ver Ploeg, United States Department of Agriculture, Economic
    Research Service
Wendy Wasserman, Farmers Market Coalition
John Weidman, The Food Trust
Neil Wrigley, University of Southampton, UK